A Horseman's Handbook

Peter Rossdale M.A., F.R.C.V.S.

Horse Ailments Explained

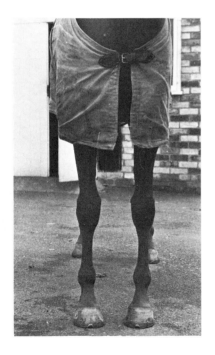

Arco Publishing Company, Inc.
New York

Title page A two-year-old racehorse showing bad conformation of the fore-limbs. Note how the toes turn in. Nonetheless this filly won races.

Acknowledgements

The author wishes to thank those who assisted in the preparation of the subjects for photography that are included in the illustrations in this book: In particular
Alan Baker
David Bartle
A. W. (Bill) Johnson
Patrice Nicol
Masayoshi Sugahara
John Vaughan
Alan and Judith Walker
John and Phillipa Winter

Line illustrations drawn
by Michael Hunt

I am deeply indebted to my colleagues in practice, Michael Hunt, Colin Peace, Raymond Hopes, Sidney Ricketts and Nicholas Wingfield-Digby for their support which enabled me to write this book.

I am very grateful to Sue Ellis who typed the manuscript and without whose help this book would not have been possible.

First published in Great Britain in 1979
by Ward Lock Limited, a Pentos Company.

Published 1979 by Arco Publishing
Company, Inc. 219 Park Avenue South,
New York, N.Y. 10003

Library of Congress Cataloging in
Publication Data
Rossdale, Peter D.
   Horse ailments explained.
   (A Horseman's handbook)
   1. Horses—Diseases. I. Title. II. Series.
SF951.R72   636.1'08'97   78-8941
ISBN 0-668-04582-5
ISBN 0-668-04586-8 pbk.

Printed in Great Britain by
T. & A. Constable Ltd, Edinburgh

Contents

Introduction

This book is about the ailments of horses. Its object is to help you, the owner, rider, groom or onlooker, to gain a better understanding of the horse in health and illness. If, for example, your horse has a swollen leg or a 'snotty' nose you will be better able to appreciate their significance in relation to what is actually happening to the horse.

But this book is not designed as a do-it-yourself guide to amateur diagnosis and home remedies. You should hold your horse, any horse, in greater esteem than to come between it and those professionally qualified to attend to its needs in ill health. It has been truly said that a little knowledge is a dangerous thing, and nowhere is this more true than in medicine. We may 'doctor' ourselves from time to time, but that is our responsibility. It is a foolish parent who administers to his or her child without at least consulting a doctor.

The professional man or woman is trained to diagnose and treat and, from experience, to avoid the mistakes which may be made by the untrained person. I therefore make no apologies for the fact that within the pages of this book you will repeatedly find the advice 'consult your vet'. But vets, like doctors, are busy people and will not want to visit your horse unnecessarily. The vet/client relationship should be based on mutual trust — the client having confidence that his vet will do his or her best but not incur unnecessary expense; the vet that the client will seek advice before treating a case and not jeopardize it through negligence in carrying out the measures recommended.

Your vet

Your vet provides a service twenty-four hours of each day, 365 days of the year. He, or one of his colleagues, will always be available to speak to you or, when necessary, to attend your horse.

Practising vets do not, indeed cannot, have a nine to five mentality. But just like you, the reader, they have to organize their lives along reasonable lines, so bear in mind the following:

(*a*) If you want a visit phone the surgery soon after it has opened in the morning.

(*b*) Make plain to whoever takes the message whether or not the matter is urgent. There is all the difference between a horse showing signs of colic, and one that has had a sore on its skin for several days. Both cases need attention, but one urgently and the other could wait another twenty-four hours.

(*c*) If you only want advice, find out from the secretary during office hours when you should phone your vet, or leave a message asking him to phone you at his convenience. Do not, unless absolutely essential, phone him at home during meal-times or late at night. Be brief when speaking to him on the phone — other people may be trying to reach him!

(*d*) Call your vet at as early a stage as possible. He would rather see a case too early than too late.

(*e*) Do not employ remedies of your own or those that have been prescribed for previous cases before obtaining your vet's approval. You can harm your horse by using the wrong remedy or by delaying treatment. An extreme example of this is the owner who treats the wound on a horse for two weeks and then calls the vet just before the horse develops lockjaw.

(*f*) Make a note of any symptoms that you observe and report them concisely and accurately. Be prepared to provide your vet with an outline of the horse's veterinary history.

(*g*) Do not deliberately hold back information about the case (you may have caused an injury, inadvertently administered a noxious substance, forgotten to provide water or used a home remedy that has gone wrong). You can trust your vet to be discreet and treat all that you tell him in confidence.

(*h*) Do not try to prove to your vet that you are better than he at diagnosing and treating — he is trained in science and you are not. However, there is every reason why you should discuss a case with your vet and thereby learn the whys and wherefores of his diagnosis and treatment. If you feel you would like a second opinion you should only have to ask and your vet will suggest the best person for the particular case.

One of the most important don'ts is DON'T consult other vets or experts behind your own vet's back. This — if you will forgive the pun — may rightly put his back up, and it is a dangerous habit because you will eventually find you have no professional as a friend.

Vets also ask for your indulgence should they be unpunctual. A daily round may be disrupted by an emergency call, a case may take longer than anticipated or, as often happens, a client may present more cases than expected ('Could you just have a look at this one — it has a six-inch gash on its leg that needs stitching!'). Once when I apologized to a client for being late he replied 'You're not late unless you don't turn up!' This, I feel, is rather an understanding attitude to take, don't you agree? However, vets do realize the difficulties caused to staff by unpunctuality when it happens to them, so you will usually find him sympathetic if he himself is consistently late. This, of course, is what the vet/client relationship is all about — a capacity for mutual understanding.

Take an opportunity to discuss all ailments with your vet; find out what measures you should take in an emergency, and how to manage a sick or injured horse.

1 Knowing the signs of health

We must be able to recognize the signs of health before we can learn to interpret those of ill health.

Recognizing a healthy horse is partly intuitive. Anyone who has fed, watered and generally cared for horses often instinctively knows when they are unwell. Here a knowledge of the individual horse is all-important, and thus we hear people say that they knew Dobbin was ill as soon as they opened the box door because 'he didn't whinny as he usually does'. In this case the person knew the habits of Dobbin and deduced the absence of the whinny to be a sign of ill health. Vets use this intuitive sense but it is based on a whole multitude of signs, from behaviour to the way the horse moves, eats and passes dung. Vets are trained to observe these signs, but there is no reason why the novice horse-handler should not acquire the skill. Let us examine the horse's functions in more detail and perhaps acquire the intuition of Dobbin's owner.

Behaviour is part habit, part instinct and part a response to happenings in the horse's surroundings. For example, a horse comes to the gate at 3 p.m. because that is the time it is fed, a car backfires, and instinctively the horse gallops to the centre of the field. There the horse sees the familiar figure of its owner, hears a reassuring voice and smells the oats held in an outstretched hand. Reacting to these 'stimuli' he allows himself to be caught. A knowledge of the individual is therefore important because a high-spirited horse that is easily caught may be exhibiting signs of ill health.

Feeding

Horses feed out of habit, demanding at times and refusing at others. In nature the horse is a continuous feeder, but the way it is usually managed entails that it is at times short of food, and at others has it in abundance. Although the horse adapts to this irregular feeding programme it nevertheless has its own inherent rhythm of feeding and resting. Thus a horse which is continuously at pasture will have periods of grazing, exercise and rest. At the end of a grazing period the horse will refuse grass but it may eat titbits or corn, not from hunger but as a change from grass. Similarly a horse stabled for twenty-four hours will usually eat grass when this is offered. Refusal to feed usually indicates ill health especially in the digestive system. It may be helpful to offer the horse a tempting handful of corn or grass to see if it has any appetite.

The manner of eating is an important guide to the health of areas such as the tongue, teeth, pharynx (back of the throat) and gullet — those parts involved in mastication and swallowing. A horse normally uses its lips to bring food between the front teeth, which are used for cutting, so that the tongue can convey relatively small pieces of food to the cheek teeth. These act as millstones, grinding the food into a bolus mixed with saliva, which is then carried by the tongue into the gullet and thence propelled to the stomach. The whole process, from lips to stomach, takes place in a remarkably orderly fashion. It is only when a part of the mechanism is damaged that we can really appreciate the smooth and efficient way the horse eats its food. A cut gum, painful tooth, sore pharynx or blocked gullet lead to signs of cudding (dropping pledgelets of food), irregular chewing movements and drooling saliva.

The horse's approach to drinking is similar to the habits of eating — a little and often. Should water not be readily available this pattern may be altered and large draughts taken infrequently. Normally when a horse drinks it does so with deliberate movements and does not linger in its action. A horse which swills water slowly through the mouth is probably suffering from some digestive upset, whereas one that stands with its head hanging over the water manger may be suffering from 'choke' (see p. 13) or some other chronic obstruction of the alimentary tract.

The quantity of water drunk varies according to the age and size of horse, type of feed, surrounding temperature and amount of exercise taken. Thus individual requirements vary from 22·75-90·90 l (5-20 gal) a day, and it is not possible to state categorically that a horse is drinking too little or too much merely by measuring its daily consumption. If the horse appears healthy in all respects, eats normally and passes dung of reasonable size and consistency, it may be judged to be drinking sufficiently for its needs, whatever its intake. If it suddenly increases or decreases its consumption then we may suspect either a change in management (for example, the amount of salt being fed) or change in an internal function, which may possibly be the result of some disease.

Digestion

You will have seen how the amount of, and manner in which food and water are consumed helps you to judge the health of your horse. In the same way, you should observe the amount and consistency of waste material, urine and faeces, excreted. First let us consider defaecation.

The consistency of the dung, from sloppy cow-like droppings to hard small pellets, depends on the amount of water it contains. This in turn is related to a number of different factors. For example, the rate at which food is propelled down the digestive tract significantly alters the amount of water that is left in the faeces, thus when the gut is over-active, as in diarrhoea or when the horse is excited, the dung is soft or fluid, and if the gut is relatively sluggish the dung becomes dry and firm. The nature of the food can also determine the consistency of the dung, a fact illustrated by the difference we expect to find in horses on spring pastures compared with those on a diet of hay and corn. The difference is due partly to the water content of the diet and partly to the nature (proportion of fibre, protein and so on) of the food. The horse digests the fibre by means of the bacteria in the large colon, and these bacteria alter according to the particular food. Some foods, and substances such as antibiotics, may induce the wrong kind of bacteria to flourish and lead to very soft, high-smelling dung.

A horse of 500 kg (1100 lb) will pass about 20 kg (44 lb) of moist dung, and a rough guide to the quantity of dung an individual horse will pass in twenty-four hours is about a twenty-fifth of its body weight. Thus a pony of 14 hands weighing 181·45 kg (400 lb) will produce about 3·65 kg (8 lb) of dung a day.

The output of urine is similarly controlled by circumstances of management and diet. On average an adult horse of 15 to 16 hands passes about 5 litres (1 gal) of urine in twenty-four hours. In practice it is difficult to assess the quantity of urine voided because, unlike dung, it cannot readily be collected and measured. Usually, unless a sample is collected into a container, the stableman has only an impression of the colour and smell. The colour is due to substances known as urochromes which become more diluted the larger the quantity of urine. Thus pale urine indicates an increased output, and conversely, when the urine is dark it suggests a reduced output.

Fillies and colts adopt a characteristic stance when urinating. In ill health, and especially when the horse feels pain as a result of an injury to its back or an inflamed bladder or urinary duct, the horse may appear uncomfortable when staling, repeatedly adopting the urinating position and dribbling small amounts of urine from the penis or vagina. Horses with impacted colic (see p. 19) often maintain the staling stance for long periods owing to a full colon pressing into their pelvic outlet.

Movement

Every position and movement of the body tells a story. The head held high, ears pricked or rotating, and we know the horse is on the alert for signs or sounds of danger. If the horse has its head down and is grazing we can sense its state of tranquillity.

Horses make signals to one another, snorting, whinnying, putting the ears back, raising the tail, pawing the ground and so on, and we can interpret these if we take the trouble to study their habits and behavioural patterns. We can come to recognize whether a horse is pawing the ground through frustration, inquisitiveness or colic; if the horse is lying down we must be able to tell if it is resting, suffering from abdominal pain or, if an in-foal mare, about to deliver a foal.

Understanding movement is very important. To know that the horse is lame we must first recognize the smooth, even rhythm of its head, neck, body and limbs in health. This can only be appreciated by watching normal healthy horses walking and trotting, noticing the carriage of the head and symmetrical movements of hind quarters and limbs.

A horse normally gets to its feet by stretching its front legs out and raising the fore parts followed by the hind parts, and it lies down by lowering the fore and then the hind quarters. Awkwardness or difficulty in getting up and down or repeated changes of position may indicate pain or disability.

Body temperature

The body temperature may be assessed by a thermometer inserted through the anus into the rectum. Rectal temperature is a guide to body temperature, although its accuracy may be affected by conditions such as gas in the rectum and relaxation of the anal ring which occurs during diarrhoea. The normal temperature is 37°-38°C (99°-101°F). It is important not to take a temperature too soon after a horse has been exerting himself as it takes some time to return to normal.

Breathing

The rate of breathing may be timed by movements of the chest or nostrils. The rate in adult horses is about twelve breaths per minute when the horse is quiet and at rest. The rate may be increased by excitement or, of course, exercise. The breathing movements may be observed by watching the line at the union of the chest with the abdominal wall. The movements are normally very shallow and consist of a slow outward movement of inspiration and a rather more rapid expiration.

2 The alimentary tract and the urinary system

The alimentary tract (also called the gut, intestines or bowel) is a tube which actually runs the length of the body from the mouth to the anus. Every different section of it is modified for its own particular role in the process of digestion, that is, converting foodstuffs into substances capable of being absorbed into the blood stream and used by the body for energy and tissue-building purposes. The digestive process starts in the mouth where the front teeth grasp, and the molars grind, the food. From here the gullet conveys it to the stomach, thence to the intestines, caecum and large colon, and it is here that the greatest part of digestive activity takes place. The horse is peculiar in this respect, as in most other animals this activity is largely confined to the stomach and intestine. Also, unlike many other mammals, such as ourselves, dogs and cats, bacteria play a large part in the horse's digestive process. They live in the caecum and large colon, which are voluminous compared

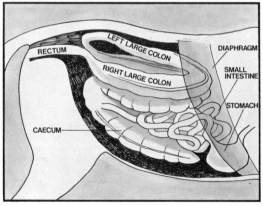

The digestive tract.

to the size of the stomach. Here they ferment the cellulose and fibre (these being found in high proportion in the horse's natural diet) producing chemical substances known as free fatty acids. These, being absorbed into the blood stream, can be converted into protein, sugars and fat.

From the back of the throat to the anus the tube has muscular walls which contract in waves so that the contents of the gut are propelled towards the rectum in a normally regular and steady way. These waves of muscular contraction are known as peristalsis. When the gut movement is sluggish the bowel contents become dry due to overmuch water being absorbed and a stoppage may result. When movement is overactive the opposite, diarrhoea, occurs as less water is absorbed.

Choke

Choke results from the gullet becoming blocked with dry food or a 'foreign body' such as a piece of wood chewed from a fence. The horse shows signs of a profuse discharge from both nostrils, refuses food and may stand with its head over a bucket of water swilling it through its mouth. The condition is sometimes mistaken for strangles (p. 92), an infectious disease in which a catarrhal discharge drains down the nostrils.

Choke may be cured by injecting a tranquillizer or similar drug which relaxes the gullet so that the obstruction can pass into the stomach. If you do suspect choke you should call your vet immediately.

Colic

By far the most common condition affecting the gut of the horse is colic. Colic means the type of pain which arises from one of the muscular tubes of the body. Renal (kidney) and biliary (bile duct) colic are familiar conditions in humans but horses rarely suffer from these forms of colic and the term nearly always refers to the abdominal pain caused by a disturbance in the gut.

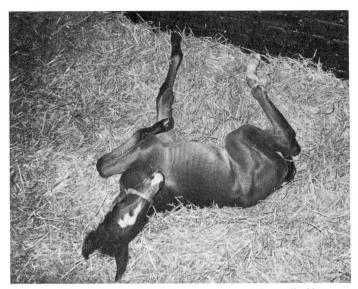

A foal showing evidence of abdominal pain due to meconium colic. Note the position of the head.

As can be seen on page 19, colic can present in many different ways and in various degrees of gravity. When a horse feels pain of any kind its behaviour alters in some way. The behaviour of a horse with colic varies with the type and severity of the pain (sharp, dull, continuous or intermittent), the site of origin (stomach, intestine, colon and so on) and the possible presence of side-effects. For example, when a mass of dry food accumulates in the colon causing a stoppage the horse feels a dull pain and will alternate between lying flat out and resting on its brisket. From time to time it will look round at its flanks and sometimes groan. In contrast, a horse suffering from a 'twist' will sweat profusely, roll violently, lie on its back with its feet in the air and eventually pass into a state of shock, displaying signs of depression and circulatory collapse and finally, if left untreated, will die.

To discover how this pain originates, we must look at the structure of the gut. The canal is made up of three layers — an

14

inner lining of mucous membrane containing the glands and small blood vessels, a middle layer of muscle and an outer layer of peritoneum, a fine membrane which lines the abdomen and in which the gut is suspended in a sheet of double thickness known as the mesentery. This sheet carries the large blood vessels, along with nerves and lymph vessels, from the aorta. The peritoneum contains special nerve endings which are sensitive to pain which is felt by the horse when they become stretched. Stretching may be caused by gas collecting in the gut and distending the walls — a condition known as tympany. It may also occur when the peritoneum surrounding the gut or in the mesentery becomes inflamed, and when the gut is over-active, painful spasms of the muscle causing stretching, as in the so-called spasmodic colic associated with diarrhoea.

The diagnosis of colic

The signs of colic are quite typical but one important symptom, present in all cases, is the refusal of the horse to feed. If a horse eats it is unlikely to be suffering from colic, but of course not all horses that refuse feed are suffering from colic. Whether or not a horse has lost its appetite is a question the vet will ask you if colic is suspected. The vet will diagnose the type of colic, not only from the signs and symptoms displayed but also by clinical examination. He will note the pulse rate and character, observe the appearance of the mucus membranes and the nature of the dung being passed. He will listen, with the aid of a stethoscope, to the sounds heard at the flank and palpate the abdomen with an arm inserted into the rectum. Special laboratory tests include an examination of blood and peritoneal fluid.

Treatment

The treatment in any one case entirely depends on the type of colic diagnosed, but the first priority of any treatment is to control pain. A simple stoppage can be treated by administering liquid paraffin and salt and water through a stomach tube — the paraffin to soften and lubricate and the salt and water to increase the moisture in the overdried gut content. In cases of spasmodic colic anti-fermentative drugs are given, and in severe colics where shock is present supportive treatment of fluids and drugs are prescribed. There are many different pain-relieving drugs now available and the vet will choose the one most appropriate to the case. Most of these drugs can be injected and so provide quick and effective relief.

Action you should take if you suspect your horse has colic
Treating a horse with colic requires considerable experience and it is best to leave this to your vet, whom you should call whenever a horse shows any of the signs described. Not only can the wrong treatment be given if the wrong diagnosis is made, thus making matters worse, but in cases where surgery is necessary, a delay in calling the vet may mean that the condition has deteriorated too much for the patient to withstand an operation. An early diagnosis is therefore essential in the management of the more severe colics.

If the horse is quiet and not rolling it may be left until the vet arrives or gives instructions over the telephone. If the horse is rolling violently you should restrain it with a head collar or bridle and keep it walking. People often do this in the belief that a rolling horse may suffer a twist but there is no direct evidence of this, and it is probable that in most cases the twist causes the rolling. However, it is best to keep the horse upright if possible so that it does not injure itself by becoming cast against a wall or dashing its head on the ground. When a pain-relieving drug has been given the horse may be left loose, preferably in a large box or in a yard, and plenty of straw bedding should be provided in either case. There is no harm in leaving water and hay available to a horse with colic — it is unlikely to eat but may like to drink or to swill its mouth through with water.

Horses with colic should be attended frequently to make sure they do not injure themselves, and you should replace the bedding which is likely to become disturbed as the horse thrashes its legs about in pain. If it is sweating profusely measures should be taken to reduce the amount of heat loss by

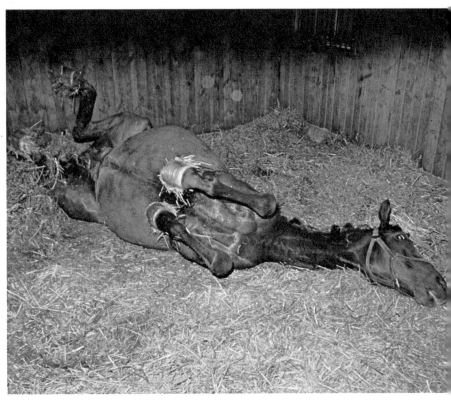

Mare showing signs of abdominal pain.

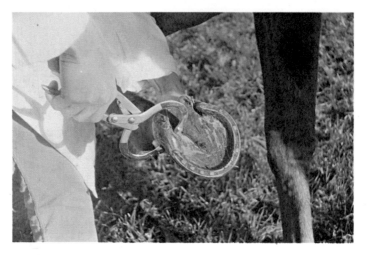

Investigating lameness: testing the foot for signs of pain when pressure is applied with the pincers.

Abrasions on the front of the fetlock joints. These are slow to heal due to constant movement at the site of injury.

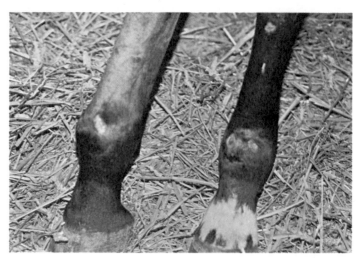

The different types of colic

Type of Colic	Signs and Symptoms	Cause	Prognosis
STOPPAGE (Impaction)	Dull pain, warm coat, sweating (sometimes profuse), lying down, looking at flanks, adopting staling stance, frequent attempts to pass urine.	Large accumulation of dry food, usually in colon and caecum. Pressure in the descending colon activates the staling reflex.	Very good — stoppage clears in up to two or three days.
FLATULENT (Spasmodic)	Acute onset, sharp pain (intermittent), getting up and down, crouching, rolling, anxious expression, passing wind and fluid faeces, sweating (may be profuse).	Overactivity of gut, local accumulations of gas, excitement.	Good — responds to treatment within hours.
TYMPANY (Bloat)	Increasing severe and continuous pain, sweating, rolling, lying on back. If gas is in large gut, distended flanks, if in stomach, belching and tendency to stretch front legs forward.	Extensive accumulations of gas in colon, caecum and sometimes small intestine and stomach due to gas-producing organisms being established over natural flora.	Unfavourable. If stomach alone affected, relief can be achieved by passing tube into it.
CAECAL IMPACTION	As for simple impaction but more severe. Sweating and rolling more evident.	Atony (slackness) of caecum, sometimes due to it being overfilled, or damage to its wall. Sand colic is a form of this.	May take weeks to clear completely.
INFLAMED GUT WALL/ MESENTERY (Infarction, thrombitis, parasitic damage)	Acute pain, sweating, lying on back, rolling.	Severe inflammation of the peritoneum and/or gut due to damage by migrating parasites or blocking of a blood vessel by a clot (see diagram)	Unfavourable. Often leads to adhesions, rupture, extensive peritonitis and shock, may be fatal.
DIARRHOEA (Purging or scouring)	Similar to spasmodic colic.	Inflammation and irritation of the inner lining of the gut caused by digestive upset, faults in diet, bacterial or viral growth.	Favourable.
COLITIS X	As for spasmodic and inflamed gut wall type.	Gross damage to the lining of the colon and caecum due to unknown causes, possibly toxins produced by bacteria in large gut.	Nearly always fatal.
TWIST (Volvulus)	Increasing pain, getting up and down, lying on its back.	Small intestine looped into knot, large gut turns on itself, strangulations through tears in mesentery.	Usually fatal unless surgically treated.
GRASS SICKNESS	Acute cases present with similar signs to inflammation, chronic cases may suffer from diarrhoea. Difficulty in swallowing, fine muscle tremors. Extreme hardness of faecal matter and stomach distended with fluid.	Unknown, possibly toxins produced by moulds.	Extremely grave, most cases fatal. At autopsy, damage to the nerves supplying the gut is usually found.

preventing draughts in cold weather and rubbing the horse down with straw or hay. It is probably best not to put a rug on the horse in these circumstances — at least until it has recovered from the worst effects of the colic. Even then it may be advisable to put straw under the rug to maintain the circulation of air and to avoid getting the rug soaked in sweat.

The urinary system

The kidneys contain millions of minute tubes into which excess water and waste material filter from the blood vessels which run in close proximity. These tubes join together to form larger tubes which eventually discharge their contents, urine, into the ureters. These connect the kidneys, one on either side, with the bladder. When the bladder is full and becomes distended, urine is automatically released from it through the tube known as the urethra.

Fortunately horses do not often suffer from kidney disease. Sometimes they are affected by inflammation and infection of the bladder or urethra, but even this is rare compared with its occurrence in other species. Stones, formed from calcium carbonate and other salts, may accumulate in the bladder, especially those of geldings, and these require surgical removal.

Symptoms of urinary disease include repeated staling, or attempts at staling, and continual standing in the straddling position (similar signs to those seen in a stoppage in the alimentary tract, page 19). If you suspect that your horse is suffering from a urinary condition, you should collect a specimen of urine in a clean glass jar with a screw cap. Your vet will arrange for it to be tested in the laboratory, and depending on the results of this analysis, will prescribe the appropriate treatment.

3 Wounds and other injuries

Horses, by virtue of their size and active disposition, are prone to many types of injury within the artificial confines in which we, their masters, keep them. A free, galloping creature is constrained by saddle and bridle and restricted by wire or wooden fencing — a herd animal with strong group instincts is exposed to enforced cohabitation with strangers. Besides, this naturally graceful and sure-footed animal can be clumsy and awkward, thereby liable to inflict self-injury.

Wounds

The severity of wounds depends on their extent, the depth of penetration and the position in which they occur. A wound may be very superficial, when we refer to it as a scratch, graze or abrasion. Quite an extensive area of hair may be lost and some blood shed but the skin remains intact and the underlying structures left undamaged.

Most wounds, however, penetrate through the skin. These may be puncture wounds which are of very small diameter, or they may be of a length varying from 1 cm (2/5 in) to, in exceptional cases, 1 m (3 ft) or more.

As anyone who has skinned a rabbit or other animal will know, skin is bound to the underlying structures by a series of folds of fibrous tissue. The skin does not part over small wounds because this subcutaneous tissue, as it is called, holds the severed skin together. But if the wound is more than 1 cm (2/5 in) long the edges of the skin will gape. The direction of the wound will also influence the degree of separation — the edges of a cut running horizontally across the front of a fetlock joint are more likely to be pulled apart than if the cut were vertical. The position of the wound also determines its extent since skin tension varies over different parts of the body — the skin on the forehead, for example, is under less tension than that over a joint. The depth of penetration below the skin depends also on the structures beneath. If there is bone immediately below the skin surface, as on the face, wounds tend to remain skin deep unless, as frequently happens, a kick from another horse penetrates into one of the air sinuses of the skull. A penetrating wound over a joint may enter the joint cavity although the joint capsule is very tough and many wounds of the knee fail to open the joint although they expose the capsule. Wounds over tendons may penetrate the tendon sheath or even the tendon.

The position and nature of the injury affects the extent of blood loss. Capillaries (minute blood vessels) always bleed along the cut edges of skin but they soon stop as the vessels go into reflex spasms and their ends become sealed. Bleeding is more profuse if the cut severs a surface vein, although even these larger vessels are eventually sealed by a blood clot. If the wound penetrates deeper vessels such as large veins or arteries, or tissue with a high content of blood vessels, such as muscle, the bleeding may then be profuse and continue for many hours.

When bleeding is at all heavy it is necessary to estimate the quantity lost. Blood is always something of an emotive sight and we often overestimate the quantity as it spreads over the floor or spatters onto the walls, issuing from a wound in what may seem to be fatal quantities. In fact an adult horse contains about 50 l (10 gal) of circulating blood volume and it can quite easily afford to lose a gallon or more without ill effect. The most dangerous bleeding is that from arteries and this may be distinguished from venous bleeding by its bright red, compared with dark red, colour and the fact that it issues under pressure in spurts whereas venous bleeding oozes in a steady stream.

Bleeding can occur beneath the skin even when the skin surface remains unsevered and a blood blister (haematoma) may develop. For example, a sharp blow or kick to a muscular area such as the brisket causes bleeding from the bruised muscle. Blood collects under the skin, the pressure prising it from its attachment to the subcutaneous tissue. More bleeding occurs and slowly the blood dissects the skin over a greater area. A vicious circle is created if an increasing quantity of blood, under its own weight, prises a greater area of skin away from its base thus creating more room for the blood and less pressure to stem the flow. Eventually the bleeding stops and a clot forms separating the red cells from the plasma. Plasma is a yellowish fluid, and when the blood blister is lanced (the best method of treatment) this fluid gushes out and the red clot remains behind attached to the muscle.

Complications of wounds
1. Wounds may be contaminated by mud or grit and are then called 'dirty' wounds. Free-flowing blood washes the area to some extent but this self-cleansing process cannot be entirely effective, especially when dirt has become engrained in the layers beneath the skin. A wound may also form a pocket on its lower aspect so that dirt is trapped under the skin, and blood, tissue fluid and debris drain into the cul-de-sac. This situation is particularly frequent when the injury occurs in a downwards direction, for example, when a leg strikes a sharp object as it is being raised upwards. These pockets are also liable to form on the lower aspects of wounds over muscle as skin is more easily torn away from muscular tissue.
2. Swelling is a frequent complication of wounds. Inflammation, caused by wound, bruise or sprain, is nearly always accompanied by filling, that is, oedema fluid. If a wound has been stitched, swelling puts added tension onto the sutures holding it together. Wounds on the leg are particularly liable to cause swelling because of the effects of gravity on the blood and lymph in travelling upwards over the long distance from the foot to the chest.
3. Whenever skin is broken over muscle or over a mobile part there is a danger that the edges of the wound act as a valve allowing air to enter but not to escape. As the horse moves, so more and more air becomes trapped under the skin, and it is particularly prone to happen in wounds around the shoulder and lower part of the neck, or, to a lesser extent, around the

thigh. The only method of preventing this is to suture the wound or to plug it with a sterile dressing and the air will eventually be absorbed.

4. Wounds that penetrate a joint cavity may be complicated by the continual escape of 'joint oil' (synovial fluid) which prevents healing as it flows over the edges of the wound, washing away the skin cells as they attempt to repair the gap and stimulating the deeper layers to produce excess proud flesh (see *Healing*, p. 26). There is an added danger that infection may enter the joint which will then act as a reservoir of infection which will spread to other layers of tissue beneath the skin. The same complications may occur when tendon sheaths (bursae) are pierced, causing the escape of tendon sheath oil.

5. Wounds that penetrate the lips or cheek may become contaminated by food, and those in the roof of the vagina (caused by giving birth) may penetrate the rectum so that dung may drop through the opening into the vagina. This type of wound

Applying a cotton wool and gauze dressing to the hock and cannon.

A sticky bandage is being applied to keep the dressing in place. Only at the top end does the bandage come directly into contact with the coat.

Great care must be taken in bandaging the hock to ensure that swelling underneath does not cause pressure and thereby interfere with the circulation. The bandage should be checked frequently for evidence of 'strangulation' and replaced daily if there is any doubt.

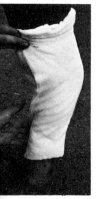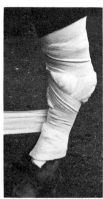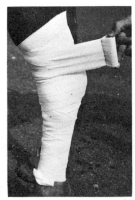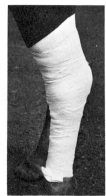

24

may heal round the edges but a fistula (passageway) is formed which can only be closed surgically.

What you should do if your horse is wounded

A knowledge of first aid is of great practical value to those who work with horses. The precise measures you should take will of course depend on the severity of the wound, the amount of blood being lost and the damage suffered by underlying structures, but the following general principles apply to all wounds.

1. Preventing excess bleeding is the first priority. In cases of venous bleeding all that may be necessary is to apply firm pressure with a pad of cotton wool kept in place by hand or, where possible, with a bandage (see p. 24). The length of time needed to stem this bleeding will obviously vary, and if bleeding is copious or the wound extensive, veterinary treatment will be necessary and will consist of suturing the wound and ligating (cutting) any larger vessels from which blood is escaping.

Arterial bleeding is much more difficult to stem. Professional assistance should be sought at once as the severed artery will probably need to be tied surgically. In the meantime, if possible, a tourniquet should be applied between the injury and the heart, but this should not be left in place for more than an hour as grave complications may result from the affected part being starved of an adequate blood supply. A rubber bandage is the most appropriate measure, but if no such bandage is available a piece of rope may be applied over cotton wool or a couple of handkerchiefs to prevent the rope cutting into the skin.

2. The horse should be protected against lockjaw which is a very painful and usually fatal disease (see p. 96). Horses may be protected by injecting tetanus anti-toxin serum within twenty-four hours of the injury. This protection lasts for about twenty days, diminishing gradually until it is lost about thirty days after the injection. They can be protected by injecting the vaccine tetanus toxoid on an annual basis. If the wound is particularly dirty and the last injection of toxoid given was more than six months previously it may be advisable to give a booster dose at the time of injury.

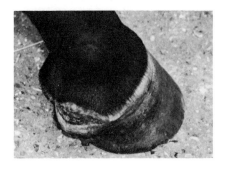

A wound at the heel has split open and is healing by second intention (see below). This wound may interfere with the growth of the hoof because the coronary band is damaged.

Healing

If the edges of a wound are brought together they will heal by what is known as first intention, that is, the skin cells grow from each side uniting the edges and healing with a minimum of scar. On the other hand, if any gap is left, healing is by second intention — the gap first has to be filled with new tissue before the edges of the skin can be united, the sequence of healing being as follows: a scaffold of special cells grows into the gap from the layers underlying the skin accompanied by minute blood vessels, hence this new growth is red and apt to bleed. It is sometimes referred to as proud flesh or granulation tissue. When the gap has been filled the skin cells can grow across the surface and unite as in first intention. The proud flesh then contracts, drawing the edges of the wound closer together. However, if the wound is extensive the edges may never unite but be permanently separated by scar.

Does the wound require stitching? The answer is obviously 'yes' if the wound is extensive, penetrates deeply or is over a vital part such as a joint, and in these cases you should always consult your vet, though there are some borderline cases where even the vet cannot be sure whether or not to suture a wound. The position in which the wound occurs will greatly affect his decision. For example, a small wound running horizontally over the front of a joint may be left unstitched because the tension on the suture thread may cause it to tear the skin allowing the edges of the wound to gape — in these cases a wound is said to have 'broken down'. If the wound occurs in a vertical

26

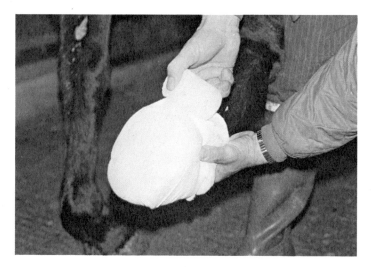

Dressings and poultices may be kept in position with a sticky bandage placed around the lower end of the pastern and over the foot.

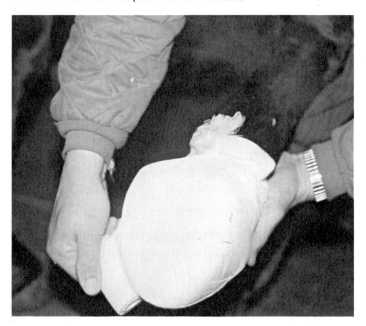

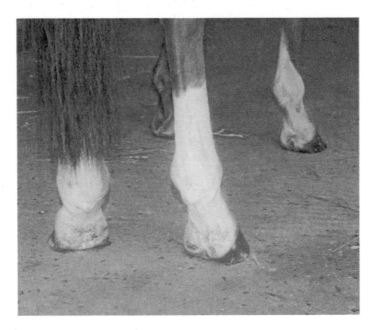

Horses with white markings are more susceptible to infections and sores of the skin overlying the heels and pasterns.

Above right Skin infections are common in stabled horses. In this case ringworm was diagnosed.

Below right An allergic reaction of the skin. This condition may be mistaken for ringworm or other infections.

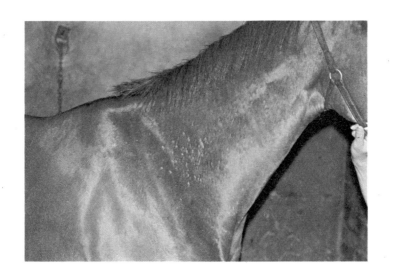

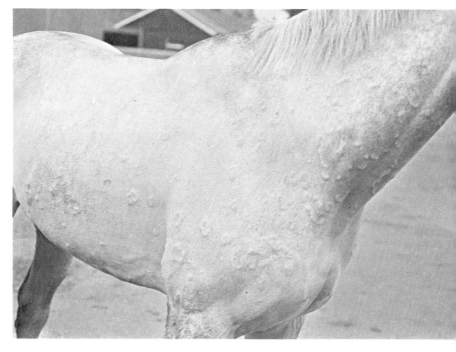

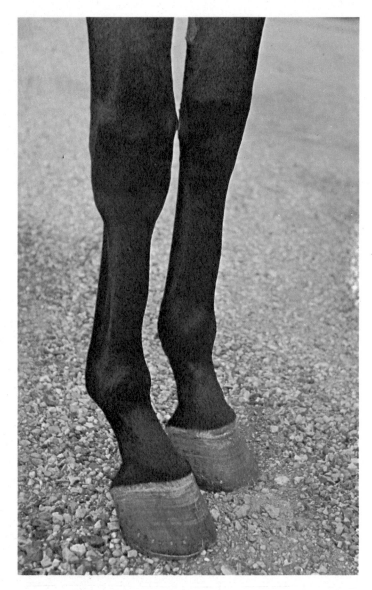

Note the swelling on the front of the cannon bone. This condition, called a bucked shin, may be a cause of lameness.

direction there is a far better chance of healing by first intention after stitching.

Fractures

Bone fractures are usually, but not always, painful. The most painful are those occurring in bones which support weight (the limbs) or where there is movement, for instance, the ribs. Bone may be likened to china and the types of fractures range from a hairline crack to separation into two or multiple parts. Hairline fractures can often only be diagnosed by X-ray, but in other cases the fractured ends may grate and this can be felt by placing our hands over the surface or hearing it through a stethoscope. This grating is known as crepitus. The extent of even severe fractures can sometimes only be determined by radiography.

What you should do if your horse suffers a fracture
If you suspect your horse has a fracture you should inform your vet. Subject to any special advice which he may give you, if the fracture is in a limb you should place a bandage or one or two layers of ganjee tissue around the part to give support and reduce movement. Tie the horse to the wall of its stall with a piece of string attached to its head collar to prevent it from lying down. If there is a crack in one of the major weight-supporting bones, such as the femur or cannon, the horse may cause these to separate as it gets to its feet, and it may be necessary in some cases to have the horse tied up like this for several days or weeks. This is particularly important when a horse has fractured its pelvis, and when this happens you will obviously be guided by your vet.

If there is an open wound above a fracture it is necessary to place extra supporting bandages to protect the fractured parts from infection and from protruding through the wound and causing even greater injury. If the cannon is fractured it may be helpful to bind a piece of wood on either side as a temporary precaution against further damage, but care must be taken to

31

protect the ends so they do not become driven into the skin.

Tranquillizers are a good adjunct to treatment and may be prescribed by the vet, particularly if the horse is liable to become restless, but you should never give them unless your vet has specifically asked you to do so.

Shock

Shock is a condition that can supervene when there is a very severe internal injury, fracture or blood loss. It may also occur in association with many diseases and conditions such as colic, super-purgational diarrhoea or infection where large amounts of pus accumulate. It is caused by a collapse of blood circulation and a deteriorating strength of heart action, and the first signs are a cold, clammy skin, weak pulse, increased breathing rate and depression.

Immediate veterinary attention should be sought, and in the meantime keep the horse warm with rugs, preferably insulated by straw to allow sweat to evaporate or become absorbed without soaking them. The box may be warmed with infra-red lamps or electric hot-air blowers. The legs should be bandaged and the atmosphere kept clear of dust. Slightly chilled water should be readily available and if the horse is lying down it should be offered water frequently from a clean bucket. Good quality food, preferably grass or hay, should also be available should the horse be inclined to eat but in most cases appetite will be lost. The vet's treatment will consist of replacing lost fluid, nourishing substances and salt intravenously, and blood transfusions are sometimes necessary.

4 Lameness

Lameness is a sign of pain and causes a change in the natural rhythm of a horse's action. On feeling pain a horse attempts to keep weight off the affected limb, thus preventing the equal distribution of weight between the four legs. The uneven action which results may be seen best at the trot, although if the pain is sufficiently severe it may be observed at the walk. At the faster paces of cantering and galloping the signs are hardly, if at all, apparent to the naked eye but they may be detected on a slow-motion film.

In order to improve your ability to recognize lameness you should first study normal horses as they walk and trot towards, past and away from you. Stand at a distance of several yards from the line of movement, as you will get a false impression if you stand too near or too far away. The horse may be bridled or haltered and you should allow it sufficient time to settle into a natural rhythm. It should be given free rein to prevent interfering with the movement of the head, and if necessary a third person should follow to keep it moving into its bridle. Take particular note of the head and shoulder carriage, the degree of sway and symmetry of the hind quarters as seen when the horse moves away from you, and the length of stride, especially of the hind limbs, as it passes you.

It is quite an art to parade a lame horse. Front leg lameness may be best seen by the horse being trotted towards you, hind leg lameness by trotting away, and front and hind leg lameness by trotting past you. In general the sign of front limb lameness is a drop of the head and withers as the good limb meets the ground while they rise as the horse puts weight on the affected limb. The sign of hind limb lameness is the reverse, that is, the head drops as the affected limb meets the ground and at the same time the hip on the affected side rises and that on the

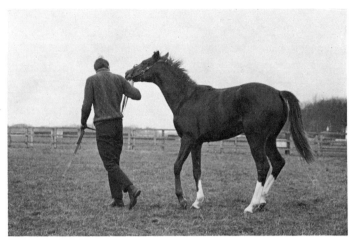

This horse is lame in its left foreleg and therefore its head is rising as that limb meets the ground. This is an attempt to keep weight off the affected limb.

sound side drops. If you know an expert in these matters, ask him to point out to you the leg in which a particular horse is lame and how he arrived at this conclusion. Watch this horse yourself, taking care to identify the alteration in movement of the various parts mentioned.

Ways in which the vet diagnoses lameness

The vet determines the limb in which the horse is lame by watching it when walked or trotted in hand. There are of course some cases where the horse has only to move a stride or two and the cause of lameness is obvious, as, for example, where a bone is fractured and the pain so intense that the horse will not put the affected limb to the ground, or where there is a painful abscess in the foot. More often the degree of lameness is very much less and in some cases barely perceptible. Having identified the limb, the vet's next problem is to establish the site of pain. To do this the vet must rely on the evidence of his examination, performed methodically in the following manner.

1. *Observation*

A clue to the nature of the condition may sometimes be provided by watching how the horse uses its limb in action or holds it at rest. For example, a horse with a damaged knee joint will often trot with an action that exaggerates the sideways movement of the limb as the foot reaches the ground, an action which is best seen as the horse trots towards or away from the observer. A horse with navicular disease will often stand with the affected front foot placed in advance of the other in a so-called 'pointing' position. The vet will also look for signs of a swollen joint or a bump over a tendon because swellings, or fillings (as they are usually referred to by horsemen), frequently appear over the site of an injury.

2. *Palpation*

To palpate is to feel and apply pressure to various parts of the body seeking to produce a painful reaction. On feeling the pain the horse may, for instance, jerk its leg away, pin its ears back or even grunt, but the vet will have to ensure that a response in any one horse is not one of habit or fear of pain

Left Feeling for evidence of articular windgalls. This is a filling of the fetlock joint with excess synovial fluid (joint oil).

Right Feeling for evidence of a thoroughpin (inflamed tendon sheath).

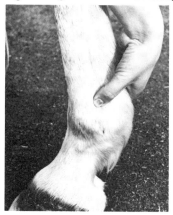
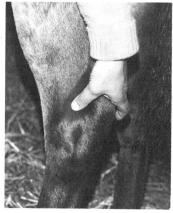

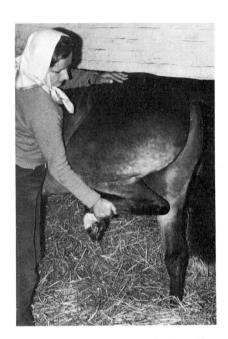

Testing the hock for
evidence of pain.

rather than to the pain itself. Some horses resent the handling
of their limbs or they may have had a previous injury and
remember the pain they felt at that time. For example, a painful
condition of the splint bone (the small slender bone found on
either side of the cannon bone) may cause a horse to flinch
when the same area is pressed many months later.

The vet usually starts his investigation with the foot as
the majority of lamenesses have their origin here. Pressure is
applied by means of pinchers placed on the sole and wall of the
foot. This test, one which is routinely employed by a farrier,
can be performed with the shoes on but is more accurate when
they are removed. If there is no positive response in the foot,
the vet works his way up the leg, flexing and extending the
joints and pressing firmly on the skin overlying the tendons,
ligaments and bones, up to a level above the knee on the fore
limb and the hock on the hind limb. The examination is more
difficult above these levels because the parts are less accessible

36

to manipulation. For example, the hip joint may be extended or flexed by manœuvring the horse's leg backwards and forwards or by abducting it, but obviously the degree of movement is limited by the large mass of hind quarter muscles which resist any degree of sudden or extreme movement. Hock, knee and fetlock joints may be palpated for signs of increased fluid content which would indicate arthritis.

3. *Nerve block*
If observation and palpation are not sufficient to confirm the site of the pain, the vet may perform a nerve block. An anaesthetic solution is injected over the nerves which run down the leg underneath the skin blocking the impulses (messages) passing along the nerve trunk to the central nervous system, that is, the brain and spinal cord, thus numbing the area below the point of injection. For example, if the suspected site of pain is the foot, the nerves which pass up either side at the back of the fetlock joint may be injected causing the foot to lose its sensation. If the horse is trotted up when this block has taken effect, fifteen to thirty minutes later, and displays no sign of lameness, the vet can confirm the foot as being the source of trouble.

Other methods
X-ray examination is the most common aid to finding the cause of lameness and is particularly useful in conditions of bones and joints. Radiography, as X-ray examination is called, is limited by the fact that although fractures may be seen immediatley following injury, other conditions may take some weeks or even months to develop before they can be seen on the X-ray photograph. The size of the upper parts of limbs, hind quarters and back prevent the average X-ray machines from being used effectively above the level of the knees and hock, and although there are modern machines which are capable of taking pictures of the spine and pelvis, the process requires the horse to be given a general anaesthetic.

Soft tissue (muscle and ligament) injuries may be more

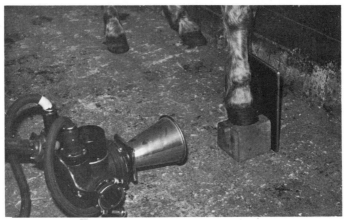

X-ray examination of the bones and joints is an invaluable aid to diagnosis.
Here the foot is being photographed.

effectively investigated by the use of faradism. For this an
electric current is passed between two electrodes, one placed on
the horse's back and the other over the muscle being investigated. The make and break of the current can be used to cause
the muscle to contract rhythmically. Normally, when this is
performed by a skilled operator, the muscle contracts pain-
lessly. However, if an injury is present pain may be produced.

Action you should take when you suspect lameness

It cannot be overemphasized that veterinary advice should be
sought on the slightest suspicion of lameness or on a sign of
heat or swelling in a vital area such as over the flexor tendons
of the fore limb or an area associated with a joint. It has always
been tempting for horsemen to treat minor injuries themselves,
but since correct treatment depends on the accurate diagnosis
of the vet, he should always be consulted. When you call your
vet make sure you are armed with all the facts as you know
them, and be quite sure to make it absolutely clear if you suspect a serious injury, such as a fracture, which requires the
vet's immediate attention.

38

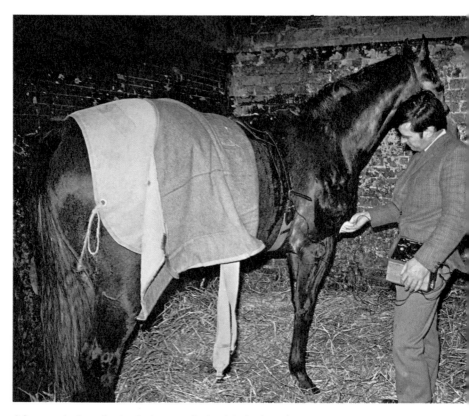

A horse under investigation for lameness in the right foreleg. The operator is using faradism to stimulate the muscles to contract.

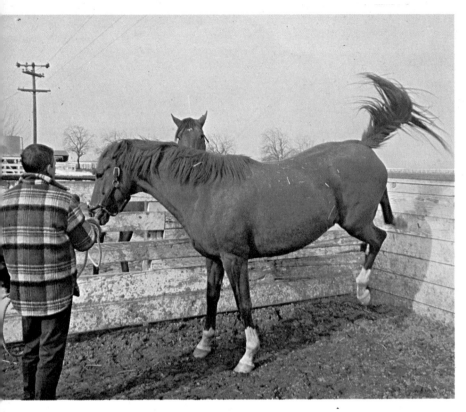

Teasing mares at the trying board is one way of determining the right time for mating, but sometimes they show all the signs of being out of heat when they are actually in heat. This mare is showing evidence of rejection of the teaser's 'advances', ears back, kicking and so on.

In the meantime, however slight you think the injury to be, the horse should not be exercised or ridden. If at pasture it should be placed in a stable to prevent it galloping and thus causing further injury or injury to another leg due to the strain of carrying the extra weight. If you do suspect a fracture you should restrain the horse with the bridle or tie it to a ring in the wall of its stable. When tethering a horse under these circumstances you should make sure that the rope is tied with a slip knot or a string that can easily be broken if he goes down.

Rest and time are the essential ingredients of any form of treatment, though often the most difficult to provide. The principle on which all treatments are based is the speeding up and controlling of the inflammatory response — the response of the tissues to injury. All injuries, whether they be strains of tendons and ligaments, bony reactions such as ringbone or osselets or arthritis in the joints cause inflammation. The inflammatory response involves an increased flow of blood to the affected area bringing with it cells capable of limiting the injury and repairing the damage. It is recognized by heat (increased amount of blood flowing through the part), swelling (accumulating fluid resulting from congestion) and pain (due to stretching of the special nerve endings in the affected area).

The vet may prescribe alternative hot and cold applications to the affected part to promote, not only the circulation of blood to, but drainage of fluid from, the area. Heat may be applied by poultice or by more sophisticated methods using deep heat techniques. It may be cooled by applying ice-cold bandages or, more effectively, by hosing the part. Other injuries respond to cold therapy alone as this reduces the amount of congestion and prevents the inflammatory response from becoming too extreme.

Cotton wool, crêpe, linen or wool bandages provide warmth and support to an injured part, though it is important to allow for the fact that swelling might continue so care must be taken not to apply any bandage too tightly. Swelling creates a tightness which in itself restricts the circulation and leads to more swelling.

5 Infectious diseases

Infections are caused by microbes of which there are three main types — bacteria, virus and fungus. Some of these are harmful, such as the virus which causes influenza. As we know, this has a marked capacity to infect susceptible individuals. Many however are quite innocuous, such as those microbes which thrive quite harmlessly on the skin, in the throat and in the faeces.

The severity of the infection depends on the result of a battle between the invading microbes and the resisting 'host'. The microbes will gain the upper hand only if they are present in sufficient numbers, and the host will be better able to resist the infection if general health and nutrition are good, or if there is specific immunity as produced by vaccination. Thus, an old, weak, malnourished mare will succumb much more easily to an infection than a young, healthy foal.

In general there are three types of infections — epidemics, isolated cases and local epidemics. Epidemics result from an invasion of harmful microbes which spread rapidly affecting large numbers of hosts. Some harmful microbes are not contagious, causing only isolated cases of infection. Others fall between these two categories — for example, the bacteria which cause venereal disease will only spread given ideal circumstances and a local epidemic may occur.

The presentation of infectious disease

An infection usually presents itself with signs confined to the affected area. These are referred to as local signs and include tenderness, swelling, the formation of pus and sometimes a mild fever. If the offending microbe spreads to invade other parts or systems in the body, the horse will exhibit generalized signs of

42

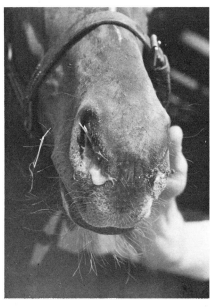

A catarrhal nasal discharge, due to a viral and bacterial infection, common in foals and yearlings.

infection such as dullness, fever, pain and loss of appetite. In a local infection of, say, one of the air sinuses of the head, signs of a discharge may be seen issuing out of one nostril. This is the result of pus draining out of the sinus and down the nose. The lymph gland between the angle of the jaw on the affected side may also be enlarged and painful.

Pus is made up of millions of cells and forms part of the body's defence against the infecting microbe. The cells normally circulate in the blood stream and are known as white blood cells or leucocytes. They are attracted to the area of damage, killing the microbes and engulfing them, together with any dead or damaged tissue. On the surface of a mucous membrane, such as the lining of the sinus, the cells become mixed with mucus and can escape to the outside; in an abscess where there is no means of escape except by 'pointing' through the skin, the abscess develops causing a softening of the surrounding structures under the increasing pressure of pus. As the pressure increases the area becomes swollen, tender and painful. In some

43

cases, owing to the pain and absorption of toxins into the blood, the infection becomes generalized and fever develops.

A common site for an abscess in the horse is its foot, where it causes pain and lameness. It will either burst spontaneously through the heel or coronet or will require draining by the vet or farrier cutting a way through the hoof.

All signs of illness should be carefully looked for. For example, a foal suffering from pneumonia has an increased rate and depth of breathing which may be seen by watching the movement of the chest. On exertion the foal may become distressed and the nostrils flared. Bronchitis may be diagnosed by signs of pneumonia plus a snotty discharge from both nostrils and sometimes the presence of a cough.

Signs of infection

Swellings
The lymph glands which drain the area in which an infection occurs will often become swollen and painful. Swellings, which are usually hot, also occur over abscesses and in cases such as 'big leg' (lymphangitis).

Discharges
Discharges from any orifice (eyes, ears, nose, vagina, and so on) may be due to infection. The discharge may be watery at first but soon becomes cloudy and possibly pus-like. It may be profuse and constant or intermittent and noticeable only on close inspection.

Inflamed mucous membranes
These are most readily seen in the eyelid, mouth and the vagina. They may be red, injected (have prominent blood vessels) or become coated with discharge.

Dullness
The term 'off colour' most aptly describes what is often the first indication of fever.

44

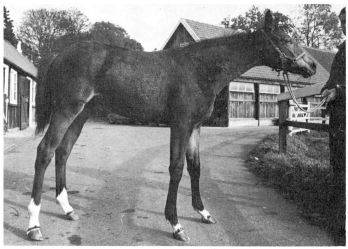

A horse showing signs of tetanus. Note the head thrust forward, the appearance of moving the body in one piece, ears pricked and tail slightly raised.

Diarrhoea

Foul-smelling, blood-stained diarrhoea can be a symptom of enteritis, an infection caused by the bacteria Salmonella.

Fever

Fever can be defined as a rectal temperature of over 38°C (101°F), the greater the increase above normal the more significant. Increments of up to 0·5°C (1°F) above normal are not considered important in the absence of other symptoms.

Coat condition

The coat may become dull or starey and the hairs stand up.

Cough

A cough may be caused by a 'sore' throat and/or bronchitis.

Change in pulse character

The pulse may become fast (greater than fifty beats per minute), full (more easily felt) and hard.

Depending on the type of illness that is suspected, the vet will arrange for laboratory tests to be carried out. Samples of a discharge will be taken to test for the presence of bacteria or pus cells. Blood samples may be taken to test for anaemia, and increase in the white blood cells and/or protein content. Special tests may be done for diseases such as equine infectious anaemia (Coggins test), tuberculosis, brucellosis, leptospirosis and so on. Virus infections, such as influenza, are often diagnosed by blood tests taken at the onset of the illness (the acute phase) and after two or three weeks (the convalescent phase). Here a positive result depends on a rise in the concentration of special substances (antibodies) in the blood related to the particular viral infection under test.

Distinguishing between contagious and non-contagious infections

Is a horse found to be coughing and feverish with a 'snotty' nose suffering from strangles, which is highly infectious to other horses, or has it merely got a 'chill'? Again, if a pregnant mare aborts (miscarries) it is probable that the cause is non-infectious, or could it be that she has the highly contagious virus known as Equid herpesvirus 1 (rhinopneumonitis) which may cause abortion in any pregnant mare with whom she is in contact?

Precautions to be taken when infection is suspected

Once your suspicions have been aroused, your first priority must be to avoid increasing the number of 'contacts' which already exist by not bringing the horse into any more unnecessary contact with others. A contact is, in most cases of infectious disease, a horse that has been in the same range of stabling or in the same paddock as the affected horse during the previous ten days or, more prudently, three weeks. Influenza, for example, has a comparatively short 'incubation period' of three weeks, so a contact beyond this is unlikely to

46

prove infectious. In some infections, such as equine infectious anaemia, the incubation period can be much longer, and a contact of up to several months may be at risk.

1. If the horse is in a loose box or stall it should be confined there. If it is in a paddock it should be taken to an isolated stable or one where it has been previously kept.

2. All material, such as bedding, cleaning tack, harness and so on which may have become contaminated by discharge should be dealt with by disinfection, burning or burying, depending on the nature of the disease suspected. For example, if a mare has aborted, her bedding should be burnt and the aborted foetus and its membranes placed in a leak-proof plastic bag for examination by the vet or transport to a suitable laboratory. Water troughs and mangers should be thoroughly cleaned, especially if contaminated with discharge. It is essential to prevent other stock from using 'common' utensils.

3. Attendants must take precautions to avoid carrying the infection on their hands or their clothes from the suspected horse to others. Special clothing, such as an overall and rubber boots, should be available for their use and must be worn only while attending the affected horse. A container of disinfectant should be placed at a convenient place outside the box where the attendant can wash his or her boots. There should be ready access to washing facilities — a hand basin, hot water, disinfectant and disposable paper towels are all that are necessary.

4. As far as is practical, one attendant only should be designated to look after the infected horse. He or she should not perform duties with other susceptible horses, though the same attendant could attend a mare who has aborted and barren mares.

5. All contacts liable to have been infected should be examined for similar signs of infection by someone who has not been handling the suspected case. If, for example, a horse is found with nasal catarrh and a temperature, all other contacts should be examined for these signs.

The extent to which precautions should be taken must depend on the likelihood of spread and the degree of risk to others. The table on page 96 lists the more common diseases.

6 Skin diseases

Skin is the frontier between the body and the outside world. The appearance of the skin and coat reflect the horse's general health, but are themselves susceptible to various conditions and infections — we take pride in the healthy sheen of a well-groomed horse and note with concern when it is rough and 'staring'.

The skin acts as a barrier to harmful microbes. It also contains nerve endings which transmit pain signals to the brain and spinal cord, allowing the horse to make reflex and conscious actions to protect itself from injury.

Both skin and coat are thickest in areas where the chances of injury are greatest, such as over the flanks. They are thinnest over sensitive areas like the muzzle which is used by the horse for touch. The coat changes twice a year, once for thickness and once for thinness. The difference in coat thickness between horses depends on the length of hair and the rate at which it grows. The growth rate is regulated by temperature, a fact recognized by stablemen who rug their horses and shut them in warm stables to produce a shiny coat.

The effects on the skin of penetrating wounds are described in Chapter 3. The skin can also be affected by inflammation and this condition is called dermatitis. This can be caused by infection from bacteria, fungus, virus or parasites or can have non-infective causes, such as chemical irritants. Allergic dermatitis (an allergic reaction affecting the skin) is increasingly common and may be precipitated by pollen, chemicals or the presence of infecting microbes. Thus a horse may suffer from ringworm (a fungal infection) which may in turn produce an allergic dermatitis.

The following skin diseases are the more common ones that horses suffer from.

Ringworm

Ringworm is perhaps the best known of all skin diseases in horses. It is caused by one of several kinds of fungus, the most common of which belong to the microsporum or trichophyton species. Penetrated by the fungus, the hair becomes brittle and raised up, scabs form and when these are removed moist inflamed areas are exposed. The condition is highly infectious but immunity does build up with age so older horses are less at risk. The infection follows direct contact with affected animals or indirectly via contaminated grooming utensils, harness, blankets or the clothes of attendants. Damp and dirty stables, especially those made of wood, may harbour the infection whereas sun and fresh air diminish the risk. Thin-skinned horses are particularly susceptible.

Horses can harbour the spores, the potential sources of infection, of a fungus on their coat for months without showing signs of the disease. They are thus a risk to other horses and may themselves become susceptible if, for instance, friction results from harness or if their own resistance to infection is lowered due to some debilitating disease.

If your horse shows signs of ringworm you should take immediate measures to avoid it spreading to other horses and to reduce the amount of spread on the affected horse. Grooming utensils used on the horse should not be used on others, but it is actually far better to stop grooming the horse altogether for a few days for, by grooming, you risk spreading the spores further over the coat. The extent to which the ringworm spreads and the length of time that it continues to cause fresh spots depends greatly on the immune response made by the horse to the presence of the fungus. The healing of the lesions can be helped by treatment and the spores may be killed by washing the coat with a suitable anti-fungal substance. Iodine is the traditional method of treating the lesions and is still very popular, although there are many proprietary treatments available. Recently an antibiotic called Natamycin has been found to be effective for treating the lesions and the spores.

Rain scald

This condition is caused by a type of fungus known as dermatophilus, and flourishes in moist conditions. It is most often found on the backs of horses that stand for long periods under dripping trees. Tufts of hair become matted together and the scabs can be peeled away from the underlying skin leaving a moist reddened area coated with pus.

Bacterial dermatitis

Bacteria, most commonly the microbe staphylococcus, can infect the skin causing lesions which sometimes resemble ringworm and rain scald. Small ulcers appear, becoming confluent (joining up with one another), especially when the hair is long and the infection goes unnoticed for a time. The scab, when peeled away, leaves an angry reddened area and this can be very painful, particularly when the scab is removed. In some cases small abscesses develop in the skin. These resemble minute pimples and they burst to leave small openings which are sometimes mistaken for those caused by warble fly maggots. The contents of the pimple discharge through the holes, matting the hairs into small scabs.

This condition may be treated by carefully removing the scabs, first softening them by bathing the area in a suitable antiseptic. The inflamed area should then be treated with gentian violet or antibiotic lotion. Advice should be sought from your vet on the best preparation to use if the lesions are extensive.

Parasitic dermatitis

Lice, ticks and bread harvest mites are among the parasites which infest a horse's skin. Harvest mites occur very frequently in the autumn and affect grazing horses. They attach themselves to the legs and travel upwards causing a rash of small scabs. Affected horses become restless and try to relieve the irritation by rubbing the lower parts of their limbs. This

50

'rubbing' is the distinguishing feature of this type of dermatitis. Mange mites, which usually affect the upper part of the neck, base of the tail and saddle region, can cause similar lesions.

Allergic dermatitis

Allergies may be caused by natural or artificial substances, sunlight, plants, pollens, insect bites and microbes. The signs of allergy are large skin weals (nettle rash), ulcers, hard lumps in the skin, weeping areas and small pimples through which fluid oozes and over which scabs form.

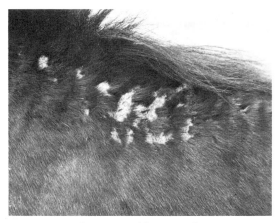

Eczema or so-called 'sweet itch' on a pony's mane.

Allergies may be caused by direct contact of the allergy-producing substance with the skin or by indirect contact when the substance is inhaled or eaten. Frequently both types of contact are involved in producing an allergic reaction. In the case of dermatitis caused by the ultra-violet rays of the sun the skin becomes moist and itchy, serum oozes onto the skin matting the hairs and causing large sores. The condition may

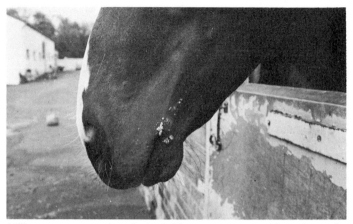

Milk warts on a young horse's cheek. These warts are caused by a virus and usually drop off spontaneously when the horse develops an immunity after one to three months.

follow the eating of plants such as Saint John's wort or a dosage of the anti-worm drug Phenothiazine. Horses, like humans, can have allergic reactions to some drugs; antibiotics, 'bite', antiseptics or detergents.

A less severe form of allergic reaction to sunlight is that affecting the skin over the pastern and heels. However, this may be caused by bacterial infection following any allergic reaction. The condition is usually known as heelbug or 'cracked heels'. In the United States any type of allergic reaction of the skin to the sun (that often results from having eaten a substance that causes sun sensitive reactions) is referred to as *photosensitization*. The term 'cracked heel' is usually employed to denote a chafed and scaly condition of the skin around the heel and posterior pastern area. The affected area may be oozing with pus. This condition often arises from standing in wet areas or dirty stalls. It is also referred to as 'scratches' or 'grease heel'. Sweet itch is a particular form of skin allergy caused by certain types of mosquito bites. It is a condition that mostly affects ponies and the lesions are largely confined to the base of the mane and the tail.

Alopecia

In this condition the horse loses hair and it can affect large areas of its body. It may occur if the hair follicles are destroyed by wounds, burns or excessive radiation or it may be secondary to dermatitis or to another illness.

What you should do if your horse has a skin disease

If a horse has a skin condition that is extensive or troublesome it is best to get your vet to make a diagnosis before you treat it. Once antibiotics or similar drugs have been given, the symptoms become 'masked' and a diagnosis is more difficult.

Particular care should be taken about lesions which appear in the saddle and girth regions. The rubbing of a harness obviously exacerbates a condition whatever its cause so if possible the horse should not be harnessed until the symptoms have subsided.

Some remedies may themselves provoke an allergic dermatitis so that, should the condition not respond, bear in mind that your treatment may be the cause of it as well as its cure!

Skin tumours

These are quite common in horses. The milk wart, caused by a virus, frequently affects young horses and clusters occur on the muzzle and face. They usually disappear after two or three months as an immunity develops. A more serious type of wart is the sarcoid or angleberry. This wart may grow to a considerable size and can break down and form a bleeding or ulcerated surface. These growths usually recur when they are removed but, unlike malignant growths, they do not form seedlings inside the body.

The skin of grey horses may be affected by nodules containing the coloured pigment melanin. These nodules, which may be simple or malignant and spread into the organs of the body, are usually first seen underneath the tail round the anus.

7 The nervous system

The nervous system consists of the brain and spinal cord, commonly referred to as the central nervous system (CNS), and the nerve trunks which run from the spine to all parts of the body. You may find it easier to understand the system if it is compared to that of the telephone. The brain is the exchange, the spinal cord, with its arrangement of nerve roots corresponding with each vertebra, represents the sub-stations to which the exchange is connected, and the nerve trunks are the telephone lines running to individual houses. At the end of each nerve there is a special cell which is able to receive or transmit messages just as there are instruments for the same purpose at the end of a telephone line. This is only a broad comparison, and in detail the nervous system is far more complex.

Nervous tissue is composed of cells with fibres of varying length. These connect to the fibres of other cells through special junctions across which the nervous impulses (messages) can pass on their way to and from the brain. Let us take an example to illustrate this: when testing a horse's foot for evidence of pain the vet uses pincers to press on the wall and sole of the foot. There is an abscess beneath and the pressure stimulates those nerve endings which are sensitive to pain. Messages are transmitted along the nerve trunks to the spinal cord where they immediately trigger off a further set of messages that, going outwards along other nerve trunks, end in the muscles controlling the leg. These messages form the end of the reflex arc that started in the foot and cause the horse to pull the foot away in an attempt to relieve the pain. This action is automatic or reflex. At the same time messages are transmitted along nerve fibres up the spinal cord to the brain. The horse thus becomes conscious of the pain and may react accordingly — by biting the vet for example! Hence the nervous system

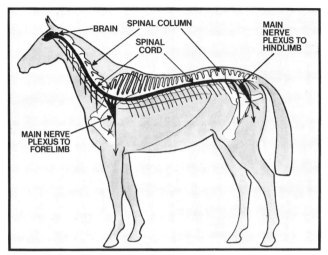

Brain, spinal cord and nerve trunks.

is responsible for reflex action and conscious control, and for the integration of all activities in different parts of the body.

Most activity originates from some kind of stimulus, as in the case of the pincers, but stimuli can include heat and cold, pressure and touch, as well as pain. The stimuli are received by special cells known as receptors, of which the eyes, ears and nose are specialized examples.

Ailments of the nervous system can occur when messages are interrupted at some point along their path in the CNS or nerve trunks. For example, the muscles of the upper lip are controlled by messages received down a special nerve trunk known as the facial nerve. This nerve runs over the edge of the lower jaw between the lower angle and the base of the ear, and is vulnerable to injury. If it is injured the messages cannot pass the damaged area, the muscles become paralysed and the lips droop, at the same time being pulled away to the non-paralysed side. Paralysis from injury may affect muscles supplied by the radial nerve, one of the main forelimb nerves.

Paralysis is caused by interference with those nerves which supply muscle and where the messages are travelling outwards from the centre to the periphery. Loss of sensation involves nerves which transmit messages in the opposite direction, for example from the skin. When vets perform a nerve block (p. 37) they inject an anaesthetic solution over the nerve trunk which carries messages of pain from the part under investigation. This injection successfully blocks the messages and therefore eliminates the pain for as long as the anaesthetic solution acts. Similarly, in minor surgery the solution may be used over an area of skin. In this case it is the pain receptor cells which are themselves prevented from sending out the messages and thus the affected area does not feel the surgeon's knife.

There are many specialized nerve cells making up the system. For example, the sympathetic and parasympathetic nerves carry messages of opposite consequence to areas such as the gut. Parasympathetic messages cause movement of the gut and sympathetic messages slow it down. When this system is damaged it may cause paralysis of the gut, a disease known in practice as *grass sickness*. Because the gut is paralysed its contents become dry and hard giving rise to symptoms of acute colic, often ending in death. Paralysis may also affect some of the throat muscles, one of the symptoms of this being difficulty in swallowing.

Another group of specialized nerve fibres are those which conduct messages from the limbs to the CNS, indicating the exact position of the legs at any one moment in time. This is obviously important to a horse which uses all four legs with such precision and power. These nerve fibres are collected in the spinal cord and conduct the messages to the parts of the brain which are responsible for controlling movement. An injury to the bone surrounding the canal which contains the cord can damage the nerve fibres as they pass through the vertebrae of the neck. The horse then suffers incoordination of its limbs, usually the hind ones, a symptom of wobbler disease. This condition is incurable. It may best be recognized by suddenly stopping the horse while it is trotting when the hind legs will slide underneath the horse so that it nearly falls. Another way of demonstrating this symptom is to back and turn the horse in

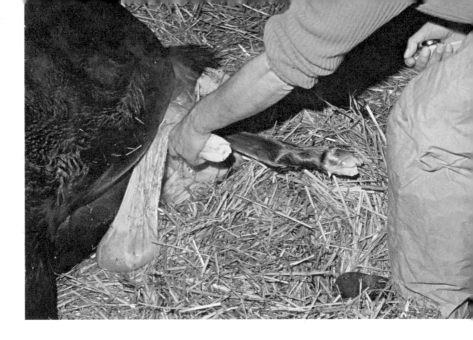

During this delivery one of the foal's forelegs has become lodged and it is being edged forward gently by the attendant. Compare with picture below, where both legs are nearly level with one another.

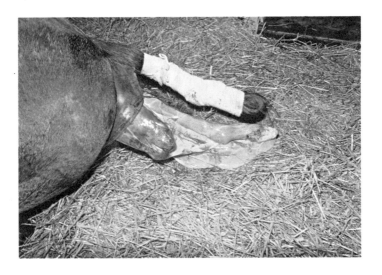

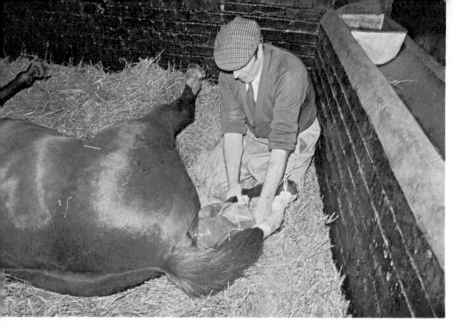

The final stages of delivery. The attendant is easing the foal in the natural direction of an arc.

The afterbirth consisting of the placenta (left), amnion (right) and umbilical cord (centre).

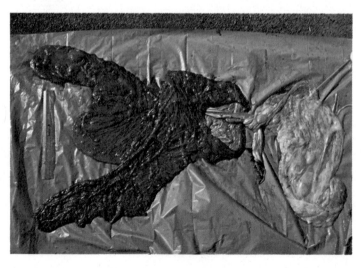

a tight circle when it will appear unsteady in the hind quarters or swing its toe as it turns.

The eye

The eye is a special organ of sensation and is constructed somewhat on the same lines as a camera with a lens and adjustable aperture through which light passes, falling onto the retina (the film) which contains special cells sensitive to light. These cells communicate with the brain where the image formed on the retina is interpreted. The eye is obviously vulnerable to kicks, other trauma-causing lacerations of the eyelids and, more seriously, ulcers on the outer skin of the eyeball, the cornea. These usually heal, although this process may be lengthy because of the relatively poor blood supply to the surface. A grey film (opacity) may cover the surface for weeks or months following the injury. If the interior of the eyeball is penetrated the fluid inside may escape and the eyeball collapse causing permanent blindness. Periodic ophthalmia, as suggested by its common name, moon blindness, causes loss of sight. The cause is unknown, although various authorities have suggested worms, bacteria, virus and vitamin B deficiency. Symptoms include a painful inflammation of both the inside and outside of the eyeball, and you should suspect the condition if your horse 'weeps' from the eye, keeps the lid half-closed and resents strong light or handling of the lids which, together with the white of the eye, become inflamed. A similar pattern of symptoms may be seen in injury to or infection of the eyeball's surface. However, in moon blindness the symptoms, which may affect one or both eyes, soon subside but may recur regularly causing increasingly severe damage to the eyeball. The pupil is constricted and may become stuck to the lens so that it cannot open properly. The eyeball loses fluid and slowly shrinks. Eventually sight is lost and the eyeball solidifies.

Cataracts are opacities or flaws of varying sizes which occur in the lens and may interfere with sight. Cataracts may be caused by infection, trauma or other poorly-understood factors.

8 The cardiovascular and lymphatic systems

Blood is composed of fluid (plasma) and cells (red and white). Its many functions include carrying oxygen (combined with haemoglobin) from the lungs and nourishing substances absorbed by the gut to all parts of the body, and removing waste material such as gases and acids. The exchange of these substances with the body takes place through the minute blood vessels known as capillaries.

The heart acts as a pump which drives the blood into the arteries, through the capillaries and back again to the heart via the veins. It is divided into two sides, left and right, and each side has two chambers, the atrium and the ventricle.

Let us follow a red blood cell as it leaves the left side of the heart. From here it is propelled into the arterial system to a capillary bed where it gives up its oxygen to the tissues of that area. It then passes into the venous system by which it eventually returns to the heart, this time arriving on the right side. Thus it is pumped through the heart into the artery which conveys it to the lungs. In the lungs it enters the capillary

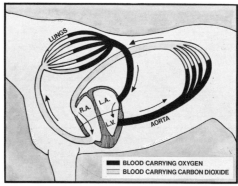

Circulation of blood carrying oxygen and carbon dioxide.

system that runs through the air sacs. Having picked up oxygen from here it leaves the lung in the veins which take it directly to the left side of the heart. Having been pumped through the atrium and the ventricle our cell has completed its cycle through what is called the circulation.

Water also exists in large quantities in the body and passes freely from the blood stream to the tissues and in the reverse direction — a process known as fluid balance. Water in the body is split into three compartments — that within the cells, between the cells and in the blood stream.

The lymphatic system also plays an essential part in the exchange of fluid within the body. The lymph channels form a system of blind-ended tubes which join together into larger tubes, eventually emptying into the major veins leading directly to the heart. Lymph glands lie along their route allowing the lymph to pass in one direction only, and preventing microbes from passing into the blood stream with the lymphatic fluid. Massaging of this fluid, caused by movement of the body, enables it to flow freely. However, sometimes excess fluid may accumulate causing a filling to develop; this condition results from the horse being fed a high-quality diet and being given insufficient exercise. The flow of lymph cannot deal adequately with the excess fluid which the high proportion of protein and other nutritional substances in the diet creates. When the horse is exercised the lymph vessels are massaged and the flow rate increased so that the excess fluid is drained from the spaces and the filling disappears.

Fillings may also occur when the lymph vessels become blocked by inflammation caused by infection, and this condition is called lymphangitis. It is particularly common in the hind limb where infection may be introduced by, say, a small cut on the lower part of the limb, and where the difficulties of circulating the fluid are greatest anyway due to the effects of gravity. The infection spreads into the lymph stream, causing microbes to get caught in the lymph glands in such large numbers that they cause it to swell, become tender and sometimes produce an abscess.

Ailments of the heart

Horses do not suffer from heart disease in quite the same way as humans. They rarely have coronary attacks causing them to suddenly drop dead, though this does sometimes happen if one of the chambers of the heart ruptures, allowing blood to escape into the sac (pericardium) surrounding the heart, causing it to stop beating.

Heart disease in horses usually takes the form of irregularities of rhythm or damage to one or more sets of valves, and we are mainly concerned with these conditions as they affect a horse's performance.

When we listen to a healthy heart with a stethoscope two normal heart sounds can be heard — 'lub dup', lub dup', 'lub dup'. A heart murmur (an abnormal sound), caused by some turbulence in the blood as it flows through the heart, can also be heard with the stethoscope. Unimpeded forward flow of fluid in the vessels (as in a water pipe) creates no sound, but when currents are created by the flow being interrupted noisy vibrations occur. However, the presence of a heart murmur is quite common in horses and many are innocuous.

The most common irregularity of beat is referred to as a dropped beat. The rhythm of the heart, instead of being the normal forty beats per minute at rest (up to eighty beats per minute in foals) spaced at regular intervals, 1.2.3.4.5.6. and so on, may go 1.2. 4.5.6. The dropped beat may occur at regular or irregular intervals. This type of irregularity is usually not regarded as being due to heart disease and does not affect performance.

Atrial fibrillation is another type of irregularity, where the first chambers of the heart beat at a very much faster rate than the second chambers. This leads to reduced output of blood by the heart and a very irregular rhythm with a rapid series of beats being interrupted by pauses of varying duration.

The vet makes his diagnosis of heart disease by listening to the heart at rest and after exercise, making a clinical inspection for suspicious signs, such as a jugular pulse wave (seen in the furrows of the neck) and filling of the legs, and by eliminating other possible causes of the signs. He will also take an electrocardiogram. This device records the electrical impulses which pass through the heart muscle as it beats and traces out a 'written' record, thus being an important tool in the diagnosis of heart irregularities.

Diseases of the blood

Horses suffer from few blood diseases and most disorders, such as anaemia, indicate the presence of other conditions. The most common abnormalities of the blood are (a) anaemia — low haemoglobin and/or red cell count; (b) states of dehydration (too little water) or over-concentration (too many cells); (c) an abnormally high or low white cell count or an abnormal number of one particular type of white cell.

Piroplasmosis
A disease caused by a parasite transmitted by tick bites. The parasite, known as a trypanosome, destroys the red blood cells, thus causing anaemia. It is only found in those parts of the world where certain species of ticks survive, and is not at all prevalent in the British Isles.

Equine infectious anaemia
This viral disease of the liver is characterized by a drastic fall in the haemoglobin and red cell content in the blood. It runs a sporadic course with bouts of anaemia and fever being replaced by periods of apparent normality. The condition is incurable, however, and once infected, the horse remains a carrier of the virus. In the United States, the 'Coggins Test' has been used to detect the presence of EIA in carriers. Some controversy has arisen in recent years as in several states the law has required that a horse registering positive results on the test must be quarantined or destroyed. This has meant the destruction of many valuable horses.

9 Ailments of breeding mares and of pregnancy

The breeding organs of the mare consist of the two ovaries, from which the egg is shed, and the genital tract which extends from the ovaries and is made up of the fallopian tubes, uterus, cervix and vagina. The egg passes into the fallopian tube where, at mating, it is fertilized by its male counterpart, the spermatozoon. Once fertilized it passes down into the uterus where it develops for eleven months and is expelled at foaling through the birth canal, that is, the cervix and vagina.

The mare's sexual function is based on the oestrous cycle. This involves a period lasting about five days, during which the mare will accept the stallion, (oestrus), followed by a period lasting about fifteen days, in which she rejects him (dioestrus). During oestrus a fluid swelling (follicle) develops in the ovary which eventually ruptures to release the egg into the fallopian tube. When the follicle ruptures it is said to be ovulating and this occurs a day or so before the end of the oestrous period. If the mare does not conceive after mating, dioestrus is followed by a further period of oestrus — an alternating cycle usually most evident during late spring and summer. In stud farm language oestrus is usually referred to as 'heat', 'in-season' or 'nearly in' and dioestrus as 'off', 'out' or 'out of season'.

Ailments of the mare's reproductive system are many and varied, but are mainly recognized in terms of infertility, that is, the inability of the mare to conceive.

Management

The physiological (natural) make-up of the mare regulates the length of time she is in heat, how often she has heat periods and whether or not her ovaries produce an egg in any one heat period. Regular heat periods and production of eggs are pro-

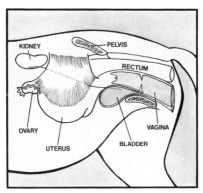

Reproductive organs of the mare.

moted, to a certain extent, by an increasing length of daylight and high levels of protein in the diet. Thus a mare is more likely to conceive between April and August than during the winter, and outside this natural period mares may exhibit no signs of oestrus.

Many mares have heat periods which last longer than the average of five days, and in such cases the timing of a mating during each season is important because the egg is normally shed on the last day. If a stallion mates the mare in the early part of oestrus, say on the second day, and the mare remains on heat for a further two weeks, the sperm (which live on average for two to three days) will have died before the egg is shed and an opportunity for fertilization will have been lost. The fact that we keep mares separate from the stallion places the responsibility on us, managers, stud grooms, owners and vets, to choose the optimal time for mating, and we have to ensure that mating occurs towards the end rather than at the beginning of a heat period. A mare may be serviced by a stallion every second or third day of the heat to ensure conception, but nowadays a per rectum examination of the mare by the vet is usually done and, by feeling the ovary, he can tell whether or not a ripe follicle is present.

It can therefore be seen that managerial mistakes may play a part in apparent infertility by, for example, failing to ensure that she is mated at the right time. This should be suspected if a mare regularly returns into oestrus, is mated by a fertile stallion and fails to conceive.

Infection

There may be obvious, visible causes of infertility, however, and the most common of these is the presence of a vaginal discharge indicating an infection in the genital tract.

The most common site of such an infection is the uterus, from where a discharge drains down through the cervix and vagina, appearing as a slightly sticky or dry material at the edges of the vulval lips which are normally dry and clean. If the discharge is copious, matter may be seen adhering to the hairs of the tail and the inside of the thigh and hocks. It may be continuous or appear only when the mare is in heat.

The genital tract succumbs to infection in two main ways. Firstly, certain virulent (strong) organisms, such as the bacteria klebsiella and the microbe which causes contagious equine metritis (CEM), may enter a previously healthy uterus causing considerable damage to the genital tract. Other organisms will only flourish in an already unhealthy tract.

Because we cannot distinguish between an infection which is unlikely to be transferred to the stallion, such as a streptococcal infection, and a venereal infection such as klebsiella, all signs of discharge should be regarded as suspicious. Furthermore, some mares may become symptomless carriers of microbes but they still pose a threat to the stallion because the microbe is carried on the surface of the genital tract.

It is therefore very important to inform your vet if you suspect that your mare is suffering from an infection of the genital tract as the significance of such an infection can only be established by laboratory tests. The vet's examination is made with a speculum through which the vagina and cervix can be seen and he can ensure that the mare is clean for service. If infection is present, smears will be taken from the uterus and cervix and sent to the laboratory for identification.

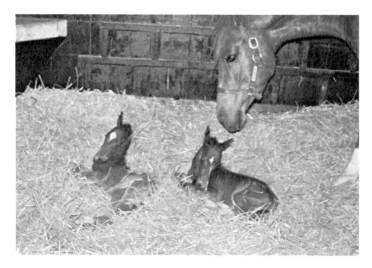

The safe delivery of twins — an unusually happy ending to such a pregnancy.

In very cold weather or when a foal is sick it may be helpful to dry the coat immediately after birth.

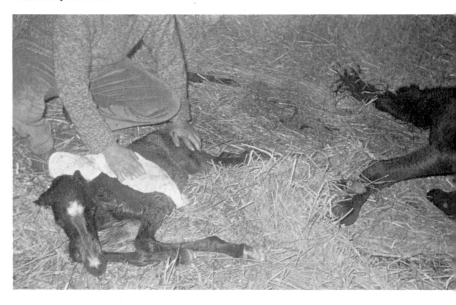

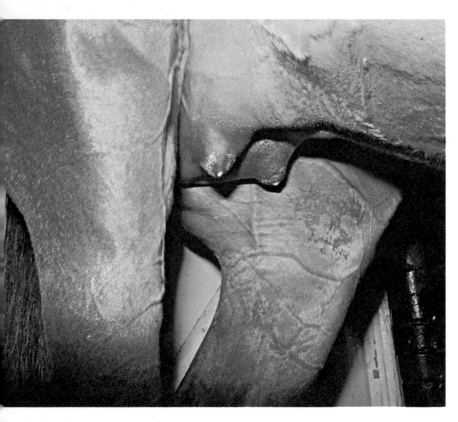

Note the milk on the end of the teats indicating that the foal has not sucked recently. Compare with picture on right.

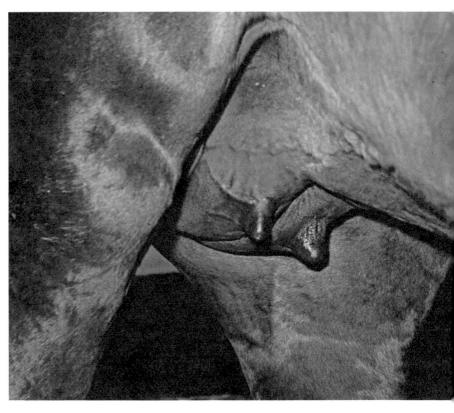

The surface of the teats is glistening and the udder is slack indicating that the foal has sucked recently.

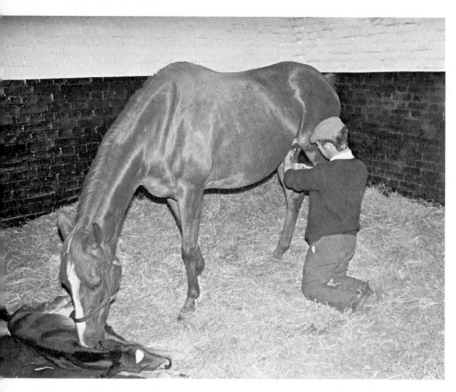

Milk is being drawn from the mare for feeding her sick foal. This mare is unusually co-operative — readers should take care to avoid being kicked.

As well as providing your vet with an accurate breeding history of the mare (number of previous pregnancies, abortions, and so on) and her recent sexual behaviour (when last in oestrus, signs of discharge, and so on) you can also help him by providing suitable handling facilities for the examination. Some vets prefer to examine mares while they are in stocks and others may be used to examining them round the door of a loose box. In this case there should be someone standing at the head and at the tail. You should not ask your vet to risk himself behind a mare that is not adequately restrained and be sure to warn him if the mare is known to be nervous or liable to kick.

Ailments of pregnancy

A mare's pregnancy normally lasts between 320 and 360 days. During this time the single cell formed by the union of the sperm and the egg develops into the fully-grown foal. Thoroughbreds weigh, on average, 50 kg ($110\frac{1}{4}$ lb) at birth while other breeds can vary from 10 kg (22 lb) to 70 kg ($154\frac{1}{4}$ lb). The only outward signs of this development are the increase in the size of the mare's abdomen as she approaches term (foaling) and the enlargement of the mammary glands which become filled with special milk called colostrum.

The ailments of pregnancy are those affecting the mare and/ or the developing foal. They include:

1. *Setfast*
This disease is so called because the muscles of the back and hind quarters become hard and painful and the affected horse becomes reluctant to move and breaks into a profuse sweat. Some mares are more susceptible than others, but in all cases over-feeding and under-exercise play a significant part in producing the symptoms. It commonly happens when a mare is turned onto a paddock, having been stabled for some days, and she becomes setfast after galloping. If your mare has suffered from setfast during a previous pregnancy you should

ensure that she has regular exercise. If, in spite of this, she should become afflicted, you should not try to force her to move but put her into a warm stable until the symptoms have abated. If she is severely affected you should consult your vet and he will probably inject her with an alleviating drug.

2. *Abortion*

When a mare drops her foal before the 300th day of pregnancy it is too immature to survive and the foal is said to have aborted. After 300 days there is some chance of survival and between 300 and 320 days the foal is said to be premature and after 320 days, full-term. It is worth noting that some people, albeit incorrectly, refer to any dead foal as one that has been aborted.

There is often no warning of an impending abortion, but sometimes, and especially in the case of twins, there may be an increase in the size of the udder. Twins are the biggest single cause of abortion in thoroughbreds. Other breeds do not seem to conceive as many twins in the first place and therefore the proportion of twin abortions is somewhat less. In an abortion due to twins one twin dies, the udder increases in size and milk may drip from the teats but the pregnancy continues with the other twin remaining alive for days or even weeks until finally the mare aborts both. The reason that twins are aborted more often than they are carried to term lies in the peculiar nature of the horse's placenta compared with other animals such as cattle and sheep. In the horse, the placenta covers the whole of the uterus whereas in other species its attachment is restricted to smaller and more definite areas. Thus, when two foals are present each placenta has to compete with the other for the available space. At best the area is shared equally and the twins are roughly of equal size with an optimal chance of continuing to term. At worst one placenta occupies most of the uterus and the other foal has to make do with a very limited area. Although this means that one foal can grow to a bigger size it generally entails the death of the other twin and the subsequent abortion of both.

Infection is another substantial cause of abortion. Mammary

72

development and running milk are often signs of an impending fungal abortion which, when it occurs, often results in the delivery of an undersized emaciated carcass with a placenta that is grossly thickened and the surface covered with a sticky discharge containing fungus. A fungal, or as the vet may refer to it, a narcotic, abortion usually occurs in the second half of pregnancy whereas bacterial abortions usually happen in the first half, though bacterial infections of the genital tract can cause abortion both early and late in pregnancy. In fact, infection may be responsible for infertility (see p. 66) and cause diseases of the newborn foal (see p. 83) as well as abortion and though we may, for the sake of convenience, discuss infections under different headings we should not forget the continuity of the various stages of reproduction. For example, streptococcal infections may cause infertility, abortion, or illness in the newborn foal and no one stage can be regarded independently of another.

The best recognized viral infection causing abortion is that due to a virus that was once known as rhinopneumonitis and is now called equid herpes virus 1. Though this is not a common cause of abortion it is the most feared because it can affect many mares on the same premises. The virus is really one that affects the respiratory system and is a common cause of snotty noses in foals and yearlings, and it is not fully known why it occasionally converts to being such a potent cause of abortion. However, when it does enter the foetus it causes massive damage to the liver and other organs resulting in the death of the developing foal and its expulsion from the uterus, usually accompanied by its membranes. The abortion is usually spontaneous with no increase in the mare's udder size. Though this is the usual pattern there seem to be many cases in which the foal is born at full term but in a dying or very sick condition.

About 50% of abortions have non-infectious causes — some are the result of the umbilical cord becoming entwined round the hind legs of the foal thus cutting off its lifeline with the placenta, but in many others the causes are, as yet, unknown. Vets are often asked how abortions may be prevented and whether such things as low-flying aircraft and the excitement of a passing hunt can cause a mare to abort, but because of the obvious difficulties in examining the 'patient' we know all too little about what is actually happening inside the uterus. In principle, however, in-foal mares should be managed with as little disturbance and dramatic change in their surroundings as is practical.

What you should do if your mare aborts

Because of the danger of an epidemic spread from a viral infection, any mare who has aborted should be regarded as a risk and the following procedures should be adopted:

1. Restrict the mare from contact with other pregnant mares.

2. Do not move any in-foal mares which may have been in contact with the aborting mare for the previous month into fresh contact with other pregnant mares until such time as you receive a negative diagnosis of viral infection from your vet.

3. Place the aborted foetus and its membranes in a leak-proof plastic bag for transport to a laboratory for examination.

4. Disinfect all areas that may have been contaminated during the act of abortion. Burn or bury contaminated bedding and wash down walls.

5. Inform your vet and follow any specific instructions he or she may give you.

If the abortion proves not to have been due to viral infection the restrictions you have imposed on the mare may be lifted and treatment given as prescribed by your vet. Any mare that aborts is likely to suffer some degree of infection or diminished function of the genital tract and she may be more difficult to get in-foal the following breeding season or even in subsequent years. Abortion is a well-recognized cause of subsequent infertility although, with treatment, many mares recover sufficiently to become regular breeders afterwards.

10 Foaling and ailments of the foal

Foaling is the most natural of events but to the inexperienced onlooker it often produces some degree of anxiety and alarm as he watches the mare straining to deliver her foal. However, as the great majority of foalings are normal, the mare being quite capable of delivering her offspring, we should base our approach to foaling on a thorough knowledge of the normal and be able to spot the abnormal in time to take corrective action.

Normal birth

The udder begins to increase in size two to three weeks before a mare is due to foal. As we have seen, the due date is about 340 days from the last date of service, but there are wide variations and some mares may foal at 320 days and others go over a year. There is nothing abnormal in either of these extremes but it does show that you cannot entirely rely on the date when making arrangements to be present at the birth. The udder size is a more reliable guide, but even here there are considerable differences between mares foaling for the first time who make a more obvious move in their udder than do older mares who have had several foals. In most cases the udder becomes distended and a bead of dried milk (wax) appears on the end of the teats twenty-four to forty-eight hours before foaling.

Birth may be divided into three stages. In the first stage the uterine wall goes into rhythmic contractions. These are painful and the mare displays other signs associated with first stage which include a rise in skin temperature, patchy or profuse sweating, uneasiness, pawing the ground, looking round at the flanks and sometimes retracting the upper lip. To begin with these contractions are periodic and the mare may feed at the manger or chew hay in between bouts of pain. In some cases a mare may show first stage signs — 'hotting up', as the stud jargon goes, followed by cooling off periods hours or even days prior to the actual delivery. These false starts should not be regarded as abnormal as in most cases the foal eventually arrives in a fit and healthy state.

The intensity and duration of first stage also varies from one mare to another. Some appear to suffer excruciating pain while others hardly 'turn a hair'. In general, the fewer foals that a mare has had, the more likely that she will show marked signs of first stage. Even the most experienced studman or vet can wrongly anticipate the precise hour of foaling, but when the vulva is long and relaxed, milk is dripping from the udder, and the mare sweats profusely while pawing the ground vigorously, then the arrival of the foal is imminent.

As the pressure in the uterus mounts and the cervix dilates the placenta ruptures and the placental fluid escapes down the vagina through the vulva. This 'breaking of waters', which may be seen as a trickle of brownish or a gush of yellow-brown fluid, marks the onset of the second stage. This stage, the actual delivery of the foal, normally lasts between forty minutes and an hour, but can be very much quicker. The speed will depend on the age of the mare and the size of her foal. It is important to note the time at which the waters break as the progress of the foal can be measured from this event.

Unlike first stage, second stage, once started, must be completed. The foal is literally pushed through the birth canal by the propelling force of the uterine contractions, supplemented in second stage by the powerful straining of the mare's abdominal muscles bearing down on the contents of the abdomen. Most of these expulsive efforts are made while the mare is lying on her side. This is the most economical position for her to be in because, if she is standing, the weight of the foal is pulled downwards by gravity away from the pelvic outlet, the ring of bone through which the foal has to pass. Mares get up and down quite frequently during this stage, possibly in an effort to reposition the foal should it be lying to one side. The final expulsion is usually completed while she is lying down.

The pelvic bones and the spine form a hoop through which the foal has to pass and it can only do this if it is aligned in the following manner: the head and forelegs are stretched out and presented first; the position of the body is upright, that is, with the foal's spine opposed to that of the mare, although slightly to one side, thus the depth of the chest traverses the longest diameter of the pelvic hoop. Any other position (for instance, upside down), posture (legs or neck flexed, for example) or presentation (coming backwards) is likely to impede the progress of the foal through the pelvic hoop and to cause a difficult foaling (dystocia).

Within five minutes of the waters breaking the amnion, the shiny membrane surrounding the foal, appears between the vulval lips. This indicates that the foal is entering the birth canal and that the foreparts are not being impeded.

As the mare strains, the two feet appear at the vulval lips followed by the muzzle. One leg is usually slightly in front of the other so that the foot lies at the level of the other leg's fetlock joint. This means that the elbows are not passing through the pelvic hoop together, thus minimizing the bulk which might cause difficulty in delivery. Once the head is delivered the mare usually remains lying down until she has completed her task. As the foal's chest and abdomen are delivered it curves downwards towards the mare's hocks until finally the hips are expelled and the mare stops straining with the hind legs still in the vagina to the level of the foal's hocks. When you watch a normal foaling notice the direction, almost in an arc, in which the foal travels as it is delivered. If it is necessary for you to assist the foal by pulling its forelegs, remember that this is the direction in which you should be drawing it.

Mares normally remain lying down for many minutes after delivery. This allows the umbilical cord to remain unbroken, and for blood in the placenta to pass into the foal. If the cord is cut prematurely, especially before the foal has started to breathe, the foal may be deprived of as much as 1 litre ($1\frac{3}{4}$ pt) of its own blood which will be caught in the placenta. This may not cause any obvious ill-effects, but when one considers that the total blood volume in the foal is only about 4 litres (7 pt) it certainly represents a considerable loss and one which, in a sick foal, may tip the balance between survival and death. The foal has established a regular breathing rhythm by about one minute after delivery and severance of the cord after this time is of much less consequence because a substantial amount of the blood circulating in the placenta has been taken into the foal by this time, helping to sustain the extra demands made on the circulation by the newly-functioning lungs.

The foal withdraws its hind legs from the mare's vagina as it turns onto its briskets in an attempt to get to its feet. It also tugs on the umbilical cord which is 'ripening' (becoming more brittle) about 3 cm ($1\frac{1}{5}$ in) from the navel. The cord is severed naturally by a tug, either from the foal or from the mare getting to her feet. Cutting the cord with scissors may produce an unnecessary amount of dead tissue which can harbour infection and it can also cause the stump to bleed profusely, making it necessary to tie a ligature of tape. The natural way ensures that the umbilical artery and vein shrivel up and do not bleed, but should they do so all you have to do is to pinch the stump for a moment or two and bleeding will stop. If it does not you will of course have to tie it with a ligature and you should always have some sterile tape available for this purpose should the need arise. Sometimes a foal is born with an unusually thick cord and it may be necessary to cut and tie it or tug it apart while holding the stump with the other hand.

The third stage of labour — the expulsion of the placenta (afterbirth) usually occurs about half an hour to one hour after the foal has been delivered. Sometimes it is retained for much longer and if it has not come away after about ten hours, you should consult your vet and he will probably remove it manually or give the mare an injection of the hormone oxytocin.

When the mare has dropped the afterbirth examine it carefully to ensure that both horns have come cleanly away. Try to examine as many afterbirths as you can so that you will come to recognize any abnormalities, such as a missing piece which is retained in the uterus, abnormal thickenings and diseased

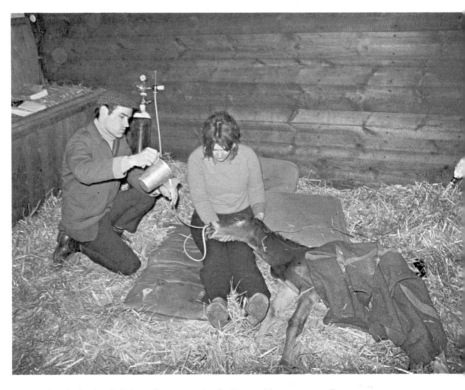

A very sick foal being fed through a stomach tube inserted into one nostril.
Oxygen is being administered through the other.

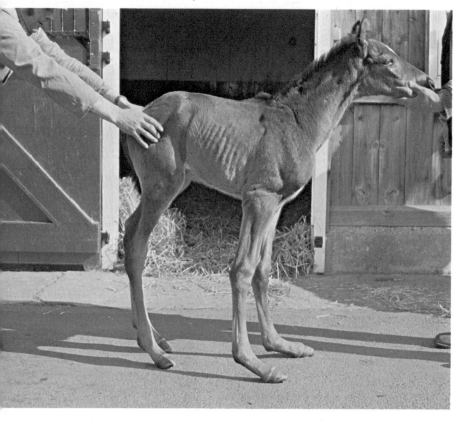

This two-day-old foal shows a weakness of the forelimbs. Simple measures such as bandaging were all that were needed for this foal to develop normally.

areas of the surface. You should also be able to spot abnormalities of the cord and the amnion. Any abnormality of the membranes may adversely affect the condition of the mare's uterus which may require treatment if she is to recover from foaling in time to conceive at the next mating. It may have some significance on the well-being, even the survival, of the newborn foal, so in either case you should keep the membranes so that your vet can inspect them if necessary.

Abnormal births

If you have studied normal births you will be able to recognize abnormal situations easily. The following is intended as a guide so that you may know when to act and when to stand by and watch, when to call the vet and when to apply your own knowledge.

1. Some mares may show little or no evidence of first stage, even to the extent of the udder size not increasing in the hours before foaling. This may deceive you as you will not recognize that they have started foaling and you will miss the onset of second stage. If all is well this does not matter but of course if the mare is not proceeding with second stage in the normal way it may be that there is a defect, such as a tear, in her uterine wall. On the other hand, some mares run milk, thereby losing their colostrum, hours or even days before foaling and the foal, once born, is denied the valuable protective substances it contains. If possible you should keep a supply of deep-frozen colostrum to give the foal during the first three hours after birth to counteract this reduction. If you are not in the fortunate position of having easy access to supplies, your vet may be able to help you by approaching another of his clients on your behalf. With or without donor colostrum, your vet may consider it appropriate to prescribe a course of antibiotics for the foal during its first week of life.

2. If the amnion does not appear at the vulval lips within five or ten minutes of the onset of second stage you should suspect some postural abnormality of the forelegs or head. However,

an experienced person should routinely feel for these parts and, if they cannot be felt, explore further. It may be that you are able to diagnose and correct a malposture but, remembering that time is short and speed of the essence, you may prefer to phone your vet and ask him to come immediately. The vet will not mind arriving to find that in fact all is well, especially if the foal has been safely delivered.

3. A difficult decision to be made is how much pull, if any, should be applied to the forelegs during delivery, and the ability to judge this comes with experience. Once the muzzle and forelegs have emerged you should watch the mare and observe how much force she is herself exerting. Some mares strain quite violently while others, particularly older mares, give the impression that they are waiting for you to pull the foal from them. Be guided by the fact that gentle pulling can do no harm provided the mare assists by straining as you pull, and the direction of the pull is in line with the arc the foal makes as it passes through the pelvic hoop. Easing a foreleg forward if it becomes retained may enable the mare to deliver more easily. Bear in mind however that pushing, not pulling, is the natural force in birth and excess pulling may cause the mare to fracture one of the foal's ribs which is itself quite a common birth injury.

4. If you see the foal gasp before the chest has been delivered you must make every effort to deliver the foal as quickly as possible. Do not mistake the twitching of the nostrils for breathing movements as these are only reflex actions. The critical fact is whether or not the umbilical cord is under pressure. It is not likely to be crushed so long as the chest is not in the birth canal, but as soon as the navel passes over the brim of the pelvis, as it does when the foal's chest is half delivered, there is the possibility that the cord will be compressed and the foal left short of oxygen. Normally delivery is accomplished in time for breathing to take over from the placenta but if delivery is impeded the foal may fall between its two supplies of oxygen, the placenta and the lungs.

5. Sometimes the foal's hips get caught on the pelvic hoop and it becomes necessary to twist its body in one direction or

82

another. A serious, and often fatal, consequence of this is when the hind legs are abnormally flexed causing the hind feet to become lodged on the pelvic hoop.

6. You should note the colour of the amnion when it appears. It should have a white, shiny appearance and the fluid contained in it should be straw-coloured. If it is brown and the membrane is discoloured it means that the foal has defaecated (passed faeces), indicating that the foal has momentarily been deprived of oxygen, perhaps by the hind leg getting caught in the umbilical cord just before foaling. In these circumstances you should be prepared to assist in the delivery and to take extra care to keep the foal warm and dry its coat after it is born. Having helped to deliver the foal you should inform your vet so that he may take any further measures he thinks necessary.

Ailments of the newborn foal

The newborn foal is liable to suffer from any condition which has interfered with its normal development in-utero. Any event, such as an infection, which damages the placenta may seriously impair the health of the unborn foal and thereby diminish its ability to overcome the challenges of its new surroundings after foaling. It is important therefore that you should examine the afterbirth (see p. 58) for abnormal features and retain it for veterinary inspection should the foal show signs of ill health during its first day of life.

There are five categories of ailments affecting newborn foals and their signs, arranged roughly in order of appearance, are:

1. *Failure to breathe*

A foal normally starts breathing movements within thirty to sixty seconds of delivery of its hips from the mare's vagina. If no such movements appear, or if the foal does a series of gasps and then stops breathing, you should immediately remove any membrane remaining around its nostrils. Now stretch its head and neck forward and, holding the lower nostril closed and the upper nostril open, place your lips against the open nostril and blow into it until you can see the chest rising. Remove your lips and allow the elastic recoil of the chest to exhale the air. Repeat the process at intervals of about ten seconds until the foal begins to breathe on its own. If the heart is beating, breathing will probably start after a few of these artificial respirations. If it is not beating it is unlikely that you will be able to revive the foal because it may have been dead for some time.

Alternatively you can use a rubber tube attached to an oxygen cylinder. Close the upper nostril around the tube, watch for the chest to expand, being careful not to over-inflate the lungs, release the nostril and remove the tube to allow the exhaled air to pass out of the lungs. Repeat the process allowing the same time interval as in the lung to lung method. The flow rate of oxygen should be about 5 litres (1 gal) per minute, a rate which can be read from the gauge on the cylinder.

In any case of failure to breathe you should call your vet immediately as the foal is sure to require further assistance.

2. *Inability to stand or get up unaided*
The foal should be able to get to its feet within at least two hours of being born. If it takes longer you should consult your vet. This also applies to a foal which succeeds in standing once but then appears to become weak and can only hold the sucking position with difficulty. The term 'sleepy foal' is used to describe these cases as it fits the symptoms which are usually seen between twenty-four and forty-eight hours from birth.

3. *Inability to suck*
A foal that goes off suck may be suffering from an infection, when it gradually loses the strength to suck, from pressure on the brain caused by haemorrhage or fluid, usually a sudden onset with loss of suck reflex, or from meconium colic.

4. *Meconium colic*
A foal normally passes its meconium during the first three days after it is born and after this time begins to pass the yellow milk dung composed of the first milk. Some foals have prob-

lems in passing the meconium. They strain, roll in pain and lie on the ground with their head turned back or flexed between the fore legs. In these cases the vet will inject a pain-killing drug and administer laxatives through a stomach tube.

You can help the foal by giving an enema of warm soapy water or a syringe full of warm liquid paraffin into the rectum, and the best time to do this is just after it has sucked for the first time. It should not be done too often as it is inclined to cause ballooning of the rectum which will make it even more difficult for the foal to pass the dung. The tube you insert into the rectum should be soft (rubber or plastic) and free from any sharp edges. Never force it against an obstruction — remember that you can harm the rectum and the anus by rough handling and it is possible to rupture the rectum, so be gentle and patient. The temperature of the paraffin or water should not be more than blood heat. If you are in any doubt ask someone more experienced to show you the correct technique.

5. *Jaundice*

Haemolytic jaundice is a comparatively rare disease. The signs, which are usually seen when the foal is twenty-four hours old, are rapid breathing and a fast heart rate, especially on exertion. Jaundice on the whites of the eyes and on the lining of visible membranes, such as those in the mouth, will clinch the diagnosis. The signs are due to a very severe anaemia resulting from the destruction of the foal's red blood cells by substances present in the mare's colostrum. Unless the cells are replaced the foal will probably die within a matter of hours, so you should call your vet immediately you become suspicious.

Looking after the newborn foal

The newborn foal should be regarded as normal unless there are any reasons to believe otherwise. But in order that you may be able to identify abnormalities when they do occur take every opportunity to observe the behaviour of newborn foals.

Here are a few DON'Ts. Don't hustle the newborn foal

before it sucks from the mare. This is a learning period and handling may disrupt the natural bond-forming process between mare and foal. Don't wear a dark overall — the foal may try to follow you rather than the mare. Don't force it to stand or suck before it is ready — it may confuse it or even cause it to go into convulsions. Don't struggle with a young foal — its heart is already under severe strain just coping with adjusting to its new environment and the effort of struggling may tip the balance against its survival. This is particularly important if the foal is ill. If the mare is very fractious or ticklish around the thighs and udder, as sometimes happens in mares foaling for the first time, it may be necessary to restrain her with a twitch. This can be dangerous, however, as it is liable to increase her blood pressure and precipitate a haemorrhage.

Here are a few DOs. Do note the time that the foal is delivered, when it stands and sucks for the first time. Watch its behaviour, how it gets to its feet and lies down, how alert and how responsive it is to its new environment. If it takes more than two hours to stand do phone your vet for advice. If it has not sucked for the first time within three hours you might consider milking the mare of about 285 g (10 oz) of colostrum and giving this to the foal by bottle and artificial teat. If it will not suck or appears sleepy call your vet as it is vital that it should receive colostrum within a few hours of birth.

Give the foal some liquid paraffin into its rectum (see p. 85) after it has sucked from the mare. Put a canvas halter on the foal's head when it is twenty-four hours old, but make sure it fits and does not rub the eyes when it is used for restraint.

Examine the umbilical stump at the navel each day to ensure that no swelling (hard, probably an abscess, or soft, possibly a hernia) is present.

Watch for signs of diarrhoea. At the 'foal heat' (the first after foaling) this may be normal but at other times you should seek veterinary advice.

Make sure that the foal is sucking from the mare at all times. When you enter the box or approach the mare in the paddock get into the habit of looking at her udder. If it is dry and swollen or a bead of milk can be seen at the teat the foal will not have sucked recently. If a foal has sucked recently the mare's teats will be wet and the glands slack.

Ailments of the older foal

As the foal progresses into its second week of life and beyond it becomes increasingly strong and independent, more interested in play, and may be found at greater distances from the mare when at pasture. Sucking bouts become less frequent and more prolonged as the foal gets older. Ailments from which the foal may suffer from a week old to weaning time are as follows:

1. *Lockjaw* (*tetanus*)
This disease can affect horses of all ages but the newborn foal is particularly susceptible because the microbe can gain entrance through the umbilicus and live in the blood clot which forms immediately within the abdomen. The microbe, called the prostridium tetani, produces a toxin which attacks the

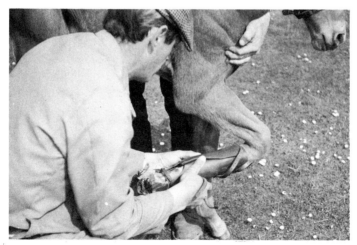

Applying a special boot with steel support in front to correct a tendency to 'knuckle over' at the fetlock in a young foal.

nerves causing very painful spasms which may result in death. The sign of lockjaw is a stiffness which develops into muscular spasms affecting the head and body. These spasms are most easily seen when the horse is lying on its side, and they may become so severe that it is unable to get to its feet. When standing the affected horse turns in one piece and has a board-like appearance with the ears pricked forward, nostrils flared and, if the face is tapped, the third eyelid will go into spasms across the eyeball from the inner angle.

The foal may be protected from lockjaw by immunizing the mare with vaccine before she foals or by giving temporary protection of tetanus anti-toxin serum to the foal shortly after birth and again at about twenty-one days. This will afford protection for the vital six weeks when the foal is most susceptible. Then the foal may be vaccinated as for an adult.

2. Joint-ill

This condition, also known as pyemia or infective arthritis, usually develops within the first three months of life. As the name suggests it is an infection of the joints but it may also cause an abscess to develop just inside the navel. Signs include painful swellings of one or more joints, often the fetlock, knee, stifle or hock, which cause lameness and the foal will usually suffer a fever of between $38.8°$-$40°C$ ($102°$-$104°F$). The severity of the condition varies from a simple inflammation of the joint, with a collection of pus in the joint cavity, to abscesses deep in the bone adjacent to the joint. It may be cured with antibiotics although, if abscesses develop in the bone, the outcome is much less favourable. In any event the joint may suffer lasting damage which will result in unsoundness when the horse is broken to harness. You should consult your vet if you see signs suspicious of joint-ill, and remember that the best way of protecting a foal from all infections is to ensure it receives colostrum at birth.

3. Diarrhoea

Diarrhoea (scouring or purging as the jargon goes) may be caused by virus, bacteria or fungus infecting the small and large intestines. It may also be caused by the red worm parasite (strongyllides westeri) or by a nutritional upset such as may follow a sudden flush of grass or feeding from a dam while she is on heat. The signs are similar in each case except that they vary in severity. Thus an otherwise normal foal may pass loose dung or, at the other extreme, it may be depressed, off-suck, hollow-eyed and pass liquid blood-stained faeces, a situation which, if left untreated, may prove fatal.

Remember that if two cases occur on your farm at the same time the condition may be infectious and you should obtain professional advice. You should also inform your vet if any one foal suffers persistent diarrhoea accompanied by a pre-ference for water rather than the mare's milk. It is not normal for a young foal to prefer water to its mother's milk, but if it is suffering from a water craving you should allow it free access to the water manger unless your vet advises otherwise.

4. *Bony and associated conditions*
To say that the horse's limbs are very important is stating the obvious. One of the most serious and frustrating economic hazards of keeping a working horse is to find that its limbs are unsound. For this reason the development of the limbs during the period of rapid growth and development in the first eighteen months of life merits our serious attention. It is essential that any abnormalities should be recognized and treated quickly.

Contracted tendons, which cause the foal to knuckle over, are one of the most common abnormalities we encounter. This contraction may be present at birth or may develop at any time up to eighteen months. The cause of the condition is unknown though evidence suggests that some cases may be hereditary. Congenital cases may be due to vitamin and/or mineral deficiencies in the mare's diet or infection of the placenta. Cases contracted by the foal have been put down to lack of exercise, excess phosphorus in the diet, over-feeding and hard ground. One popular theory is that the disease, which can be fatal, is caused by the bones growing disproportionately to the tendons and ligaments.

5. *Lumpy joints* (*epiphisitis*)

Bones grow from an active centre at either end. Thus there are growth plates at the lower ends of the forearms, second thighs and cannon bones. The centres in the cannon bone stop growing when the foal is between six and nine months old, and those in the second thighs and forearms stop between eighteen and twenty-four months old. In some cases (between four and six months of age) the growth plates become inflamed and lumps appear on the inside, near the fetlock. Between fourteen and eighteen months they appear above the knee and hock. These lumps may be tender and cause lameness.

The condition has various causes. It is usually due to the horse taking too much weight on the inside of the limb which results in compression of that side of the growth plate. A horse may become more susceptible if it is over-fed and if the diet contains too much phosphorus relative to the calcium content (the ratio should be about 4 : 1).

6. *Club foot*

This sometimes develops when a problem higher up the limb, such as knuckling over at the fetlock joint, forces the foal to distribute its weight abnormally on the foot as it stands or walks. The foot grows excess heel and the pedal bone inside the hoof becomes misshapen. Many cases are inherited, however, and some mares produce several affected foals in their breeding span.

11 Diseases of the respiratory system

The process whereby air enters and leaves the body is known as respiration, and it is accomplished by the movement of the chest which alternately expands to draw air into the body (inspiration) and contracts to squeeze air out (expiration) through a series of tubes.

Air enters the body through the nostrils which run as two tubes through the skull, opening into the back of the throat. From here air passes into the windpipe whose entrance lies in the front of the throat and is guarded by the voice box (larynx). The windpipe divides in the chest into two large tubes, the right and the left bronchus. These sub-divide in each lung into much smaller tubes (bronchioles) which in turn transport the air into millions of small air sacs (alveoli).

It is in these alveoli that oxygen from the air is taken into the blood stream and carbon dioxide leaves in the opposite direction — this is known as gaseous exchange. This exchange is possible because the walls of the air sacs, even though minutely thin, possess capillary blood vessels through which blood is constantly passing. The air contained in the alveoli does not itself pass to and from the blood but by the exchange of a column of air in the tubes, molecules of oxygen and carbon dioxide can pass in and out of the sacs by means of diffusion.

'Snotty' noses

This condition is the horse's version of a cold and is a term used to describe symptoms such as a watery discharge, often accompanied by fever. A nasal discharge indicates the presence of an infection, in this case caused by one of several viruses, most commonly one of the herpes or rhino group. The virus attacks the cells which line the nasal passages and smaller tubes

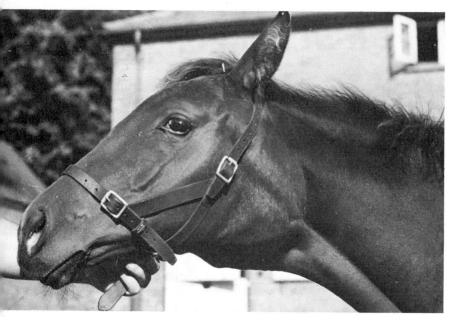

A horse suffering from strangles.

of the airways causing inflammation and thus the discharge. The damaged linings become more susceptible to bacterial infection and the initial watery discharge is often replaced by a catarrhal one which passes outwards along the tubes until it is discharged through the nostrils. The condition, usually seen in foals and yearlings, often subsides within a week or two although the discharge may continue for several weeks.

Strangles

This condition is caused by a microbe known as Streptococcus equi. It is highly contagious, causing a very profuse nasal discharge, fever and loss of appetite, and is characterized by swelling in the lymph glands draining the head and the presence of hot painful swellings between the jaws and on either side of the throat.

92

Summer pneumonia in foals

Foals are more susceptible to infections of the lung than are older horses. This disease, which is caused by the microbe Corynebacterium equi, presents with the same symptoms as pneumonia (heaving chest, coughing and high fever) but does not respond to treatment with antibiotics. The fever may rise as high as 41°C (106°F), fluctuating over several days or even weeks. Quantities of yellow or brownish discharge appear at the nostrils and the foal may appear to be 'wasting'. The condition is often fatal, and at autopsy the lungs are found to contain very many thick-walled abscesses filled with yellowish or cream-coloured pus. Fortunately cases of summer pneumonia are usually sporadic and do not occur in epidemic form in Britain, but in other parts of the world, such as Australia, several cases may appear on the same stud farm.

Infections of the air sinuses of the head

There are two major air sinuses on each side of the horse's head, the frontal and the maxillary. They may be likened to boxes which have an opening into the nasal passages which run from the nostrils to the throat. They are lined by mucous membrane and their function is to lighten the skull which would be too heavy for the neck to bear if it were solid bone.

Occasionally one of these sinuses becomes infected, pus collects and seeps through into the nasal passage and discharges through the nostril. An infection of this type can be recognized by the fact that the discharge is usually confined to one side. In addition the bony parts beneath the mucous membrane may become soft, the pus smells of rotting bone, and a painful swelling may develop over the frontal or maxillary areas.

Another pair of sinuses, known as guttural pouches, lie on either side of, and open into the throat. These are not enclosed by bone but lie beneath the skin in the triangle formed by the angle of the lower jaw and the upper part of the neck, with the ear as the apex. If they become infected pus collects in them, eventually escaping into the throat and down the nostrils.

Nose bleeds (Epistaxis)

You may notice a trickle of blood coming from your horse's nose after exercise or, fortunately in exceptional cases, there may be a gush followed by a continuous stream. In most, if not all, cases the blood is coming from the lungs and not, as many people believe, from the nose. The exception to this is when bleeding occurs from an ulcer in the guttural pouch. This is usually a spontaneous bleed when the horse is at rest and not, as in other cases, after exercise. Because of its position, over the carotid artery, bleeding from such an ulcer is extremely difficult to stop and death may result.

Bleeding that originates in the lung is usually the result of a local patch of infection caused by a bacteria or virus and is due to a few small vessels, or sometimes one large vessel 'breaking'. The term 'breaking a blood vessel' can also be applied to a haemorrhage in other parts of the body. Horses that drop dead during a race for no visible or obvious reason have usually broken a vessel and in many such cases it is the aorta, the largest artery in the body, which ruptures.

Broken wind

This disease, which affects horses over the age of about four years, is similar to asthma in humans. Symptoms include an exaggerated effort in breathing out, coughing, wheezing and distress. It is most common and severe in the summer, and where horses are stabled on straw. This is because the dust they inhale contains fungal spores to which the affected horse is sensitive in much the same way as an asthmatic person or one who suffers from hay fever is sensitive to pollen.

It is caused by air being trapped in the lungs due to spasms of the muscle in the smaller air passages. The tubes contract and act as valves allowing air to enter the air sacs but obstructing it from being drawn out when the horse exhales. Thus this trapped air has to be 'pushed' out with considerable extra effort, and a double movement of the chest made by a horse suffering from broken wind can be observed at the flank. The wheezing sounds are made because of the extra tension produced in the lung by the spasm of the airways. The condition may be complicated by bronchitis, which makes it even more difficult to maintain a free air-flow in and out of the lungs.

Treatment of acute attacks is usually successful and rarely do such cases end fatally. Some cases run a chronic course when the horse suffers mild symptoms all the time, and another type is known where the symptoms are restricted to a cough and a tendency to blow out excessively after exercise.

Affected cases should be provided with a bedding of peat moss or wood shavings in preference to straw and in the summer fresh air in a paddock is by far the best form of prevention and treatment. Most importantly, you should try to ensure that your horse is never exposed to dust, whether or not it is suffering from broken wind. Avoid using musty hay or straw, do not shake the bedding up when the horse is in the stable, and provide an adequate ventilation system. Horses that never come into stables never suffer from broken wind.

Whistling and roaring

These sounds, which horsemen dread most, may be heard when the horse is being exercised. The larynx contains two membranes (vocal cords) on either side. Normally these are pulled aside as the horse breathes in so allowing a free flow of air into the lungs. The muscles which bring about this movement can become paralysed however, and instead of being drawn aside the vocal cords hang in the path of the incoming air. This sets up a turbulence and the resulting vibrations are heard as a whistling or a roaring sound when the horse breathes in. (It is important to distinguish between noises made on inspiration and those made on expiration as sounds heard on the latter are not usually of any significance.)

The condition is aggravated by the fact that the airway through the larynx is reduced because one side of the larynx caves in and thus a whistler or roarer may have difficulty in drawing in sufficient air to meet its needs.

Appendix: Common infectious diseases

Condition	Signs
Acne	pimples or small boils in skin.
Influenza	dry cough and fever.
Joint-ill in foals	fever, lameness and painful joints.
Lockjaw	stiffness, painful spasms, third eyelid drawn across eyeball.
Lymphangitis	swollen, painful leg (usually the hind leg). Swelling may extend to stifle.
Pneumonia	rapid breathing, cough and fever.
Rhinopneumonitis	nasal discharge, catarrhal in young horses, watery in older subjects.
Ringworm	scabs of matted hair over moist, red area of skin. (Similar symptoms seen in bacterial dermatitis.)
Salmonellosis	bloody diarrhoea, fever and dullness.
Sleepy foal disease	lethargy and off-suck.
Strangles	enlarged glands, fever and nasal discharge.
Summer pneumonia in foals	cough, nasal discharge, distressed breathing and fever.
Uterine infection (metritis)	vaginal discharge.

Glossary of American Equivalents

BROKEN WIND:	heaves
CRACKED HEEL:	scratches; grease heel
HORSE BOX:	horse van
LOOSE BOX:	box stall
LUCERNE:	alfalfa
NETTLERASH:	hives
RUG:	blanket
SETFAST:	tying up; azoturia; Monday morning sickness
SLEEPY FOAL:	sleeper